Wild Life

WILD LIFE

Shinrin-Yoku and The Practice of
Healing through Nature

Stefan Batorijs

Foreword by M. Amos Clifford

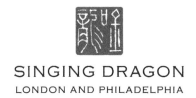

SINGING DRAGON
LONDON AND PHILADELPHIA

First published in Great Britain in 2024 by Singing Dragon,
an imprint of Jessica Kingsley Publishers
Part of John Murray Press

1

A CIP catalogue record for this title is available from the
British Library and the Library of Congress

ISBN 978 1 78775 801 8

eISBN 978 1 78775 802 5

Printed and bound by CPI Group (UK) Ltd, Croydon, CR0 4YY

Jessica Kingsley Publishers' policy is to use papers that are natural,
renewable and recyclable products and made from wood grown in
sustainable forests. The logging and manufacturing processes are expected
to conform to the environmental regulations of the country of origin.

Singing Dragon
Carmelite House
50 Victoria Embankment
London EC4Y 0DZ

www.singingdragon.com

John Murray Press
Part of Hodder & Stoughton Limited
An Hachette UK Company

This book is dedicated to all the Dryads and Tree Spirits that we have forgotten, ignored, cut down, concreted over and burnt. To the Yakshas, the kami and Kukunochi, the Jinmenju and Kodama, to Sylvanus and Dionysus, Bacchus, Pan and the nymphs. To the Green Man and the sacred groves and glades and the arboreal dancers, Druantia, Cernunnos and the fairies, piskies and sprites of the wildwoods, Artemis, Diana and Faunus, Tāne-mahuta, Iroko, and Lauma the guardian of the forests of my homeland. The time will come when you will rise again and reclaim the forests of the wild heart.

This book is also for Rafe and the future generations who rely on us now to act with urgency, sensitivity and wisdom.

Contents

Foreword

We are on cusp time, walking a balance beam. On one side is the call of domestication, of the tamed world. In that world, we can be ordinary. We can enjoy the privileges and the harvests of staid citizenship. It is familiar. It offers the illusion of safety. Of modernity. Righteousness, even.

Were we to topple in the other direction...what then? Into what land do we fall, what land that is not the tamed world, composed of all we take for granted? The road map to the tamed world provides a story of the inexorable march of science and economics, which we can join through proper education and by pursuing a fortunate career path. But this other side – let's call it 'Wilderness' – is mapped through stories. Tales we share when we are circled around campfires.

There is a story in these pages that begins with 'On my way back home'. Be alert for it. The author tells of following an inner pull. He comes to a window into a small part of the ordinary world. Looking through it, he witnesses an extraordinary dance. The dance has the shape and rhythm of magic. Simultaneously, it is exquisitely ordinary. Invisible to the eyes of the tamed world. By seeing and writing about it, the author adds to the map of Wilderness. This is the power of story.

Here is a dispatch from the beam: I lived on Sonoma Mountain in California. Often, I would take long solo walks exploring the mountain. It was not unusual to come across signs of the mountain lions that lived on the mountain. Tracks, scats, sometimes deer carcasses. I had a wooden talking stick with a heavy knot on one end; I called it my 'lion-beater', a weak attempt at reassuring myself that I would be able to fend off an attack. On one of these walks, I came across some biologists near the summit of the mountain. They were there to study the lions. I told them about the signs I came across. 'There are more than you think,' one of them told me. 'You are likely walking very near to them sometimes; they will crouch down in the grass and hold still. They don't want to be seen.' Good information, I thought. Even so, my solitary hiking habits remained unchanged.

Until.

I was driving late at night up the long, winding, forested road toward my home. I had about a mile to go when a lion came from the brush on the right side of the road into the center. It walked slowly in the same direction I was headed. No more than 15 meters in front of my car, I was able to follow it slowly and observe it in my headlights. What a rare opportunity!

The lion was a bit on the lean side, but otherwise fully grown. It ignored the presence of my car – a hybrid, so perhaps quieter than many vehicles would be. I followed for perhaps 100 meters. My inner debate: use my phone to make a video or instead relax into the opportunity to simply observe. I chose the latter.

The lion focused on something at the side of the road. It was a skunk. The lion leapt upon the skunk, intent perhaps on dinner. The two of them tangled for about three seconds. Then the lion staggered back into the middle of the road. It shook itself for a moment then continued its walk, now weaving as if it were intoxicated. Following it, I drove through an aromatic cloud of skunk spray. Shortly after the lion left the road, it went through a gate into a vineyard.

Story's not over. It was the next night when I was well off the beam.

Well after dark, I set out from my home on the walk down the driveway to retrieve mail from the postbox. Picture this: the location is well up on a mountain. The smallest parcels of land are ten acres. No streetlights, no lighting from neighboring houses. The driveway is lit from my own house for a bit, but then it takes a steep dip downhill and the light is blocked. At this point, the mailbox is still a good 80 meters away. I've done this walk in the dark many times before. I've been aware that I share the mountain with an apex predator, but that knowledge always had a theoretical feeling. Now it was different. I had seen the lion, near the house; it was no longer theoretical.

So I come to the place where the last of the light from my house fades into the darkness beyond. I was acutely aware of my vulnerability. I took another step, deeper into the dark, and another. And there I stopped. I needed to have a conversation with myself. It went like this:

One voice: That lion could be anywhere. I'm alone out here. I don't have the natural defenses that skunk has. The mail could wait until morning. Another voice: I've done this in the dark hundreds of times. If I turn back now, I risk amplifying the effects of fear in my psyche. First voice: How many times have you read the book *The Gift of Fear*?

I took the next step down into the darkness.

And when I did, my night vision exploded. I could suddenly see clearly all around me: no moon, no street lights. It was like a superpower. And I thought: 'Ah, so this is how it was for our ancestors.'

I was well off the beam, fallen for that moment into Wilderness. It felt like home. A home long forgotten but waiting dormant in my bones.

What other superpowers exist over here, in this vulnerable Wilderness?

A small coda here. I also accumulated this wisdom: when you smell skunk, you may not be smelling a skunk. You may be smelling an apex predator who was recently schooled by a skunk.

In these pages, you will encounter many stories. Each is an invitation for you to consider your own stories. What have you encountered on your way home? Have you the habit of wandering in natural places? Have you awakened from moments of absorption in your mental rehearsals of the 'then and there' and begun to notice what is right in front of you, in the 'here and now'? I suspect that you have, or you would not be drawn to this book.

So, we wander. We begin to notice. We follow instincts and encounter new ways of seeing. Each moment of true vision opens a threshold. We can choose to turn back, to the seeming safety of home. Or we can take the next step. The step into the territory where the vast and wild world waits to reveal itself to us, and so doing, to reveal us to ourselves.

For this journey we need companions. We need the guidance of stories. This book is a reliable companion. May its stories interweave with your own. What freedoms you will gain are portals into medicines you carry for the world. These medicines, whatever they are, are needed now. You, the person you were born to be, are needed now.

M. Amos Clifford
Prescott, Arizona
February 2024

Preface

It has been my intention to write a book about Nature for about 30 years, with my closest friends encouraging me to get on with it for the last 10–15 years. The problem with writing a book is that it generally means coming indoors, sitting down and focusing, and putting all these aggregated thoughts, feelings, and experiences into some sort of coherent order. Never one for dwelling indoors when the thrill of the wild was calling, I used to joke with these friends that I would write my book one day if I ever broke my leg and had nothing to do. Well, be careful what you wish for, because in 2020, just before the first COVID lockdown, I did break my leg in a near fatal freak mountain accident. After my lovely daughters had rescued me from oblivion in a foreign hospital, I spent lockdown at home, reliant on my friends to bring me supplies. Just for good measure, I then broke the other leg eight months later and was once again reduced to wheelchairs and crutches. So, my enforced convalescence finally generated this little book of musings and perspectives in service of my life's passion and purpose – being in Nature.

This is not an academic treatise on forest bathing nor a DIY manual, but it is a curious blend of mystical pragmatism, self-revelatory vulnerability, social commentary on the state of our civilisation, clamouring brouhaha over all the trendiness of Nature since the pandemic, and the colonising of Nature by corporate interests. Above all this book is my attempt to interrogate the gap in consciousness attributed to Descartes, but actually first articulated by the early Greek philosophers, the genesis of which lies somewhere deep within the emerging psyches of early agricultural societies. Our sense of separation is an illusion, a deception that we cannot yet awaken from. Our success and sophistication has contributed to that gap which has grown and become a large wedge, and we now face the imminent collapse of the biosphere.

The calls to action are building, but not yet loud enough to drown out the invested agencies of old who cling to power. To make a difference, we need not only to reduce consumption and lobby governments but also to attend to our own inner disconnects and disharmonies with Nature, so that as we become more congruent with our own wild, feral natures – so long suppressed and marginalised in our lives and replaced with candy and distractions of various kinds – we become stronger, wiser, and less influenceable until we achieve a sympathetic resonant vibration of wild, gentle power – the so-called 'hundredth monkey effect'.

The new and developing discipline of forest bathing embraces both ancient wisdom from our animistic roots and modern science and new methods of accurate field recordings of blood and salivary amylase markers. Research continues to reveal what we have known intuitively all along – Nature is good for heart and soul. My lofty intention is to invite every single person out into the woods to enjoy the positive healing effects of immersion in Nature, unconditional love, and the pure joy of being.

This book also gives suggestions for best practice which deviate significantly from ideas that form part of conventional theory in this field. I have presented my ideas based on sound empirical challenge and experiential learning over a lifetime, and, where possible, supported by other writers and observers. I don't expect that you will necessarily take it all on board, but I do hope it may be a useful contribution to a deeper understanding and respect for Nature, both internal and external.

The book is laid out in no particular hierarchical order as a deliberate mirroring of the weblike connections and synaptic threads of interweaving consciousness, or the mycelial network of communication under the earth. There are 15 main chapters, and they are accompanied by some smaller vignettes of personal observations and experiences. You can read them in any order; the main chapters loosely follow some of the themes we cover out in the woods on the International Forest Therapy Diploma training course syllabus (see back of book for details). Some topics have not been covered in this volume as they need further space to explore them fully, such as the nexus between Nature connection, mystic states, and psychedelics – the wonderful science of grounding and our place inside the Earth and the deeper therapeutic potential of this work in Nature, particularly working with mental health, trauma, and chronic fatigue syndromes. If you seek a straightforward linear narrative with lots of clear diagrams and charts and statistics, I apologise, you might find this book challenging. If, however, you are content to allow the stories on the pages to unfold, then I feel sure that this will be an enriching addition to your life.

You do not need to be a therapist to read this book. I use terms such as *shinrin-yoku,* forest bathing, Nature therapy, forest therapy, forest medicine, and ecotherapy interchangeably (they all amount to the same thing with minor variations in focus, outcome, and approach), but the desire to be in the wild is the main thrust of this work. If you just want to open a book and have all the answers laid out for you, this book may disappoint as it asks you to participate, to take your time 'to learn from the things', to just sit still and watch and absorb the 'affordances' of Nature. I don't want to be too prescriptive – that would spoil the fun; occasionally, I will be clear about practices and methods, but I do believe that we all bring our unique ways to access and liberate deeper knowledge within Nature, and potentially guide and support others to find that truth in their lives too.

Many of the themes are linked and they crop up in different chapters; sometimes I repeat certain phrases where their applications may vary or be perceived in a different context. I also find repetition helps with embodying a concept. Please feel free to question, and to reject anything that you don't feel comfortable with or that doesn't sit well with you. Sometimes I double back on myself, contradict my own theories, and offer paradoxical explanations; such are the conundrums and enigmas of Nature, and the elusive yet enticing quality of the wild.

Writing a book is a very bold and responsible way of conveying some element or quality of perceived truth, of baring your soul, of placing one's heart and mind into the public consciousness forever after. It can never be perfect, and may undergo many revisions and editions, but with good intention it seeks to move us forward towards compassion, forbearance, sensitivity, wisdom, and care.

Our own self-abandonment is surely a reflection of how complex and confusing our lives have become – we cannot attend to our own needs, or, more accurately, listen attentively to our inner self, our body voice, our wild, playful, accessible, free, animal self. No wonder we find it difficult to listen to Nature, when the nature within is rejected or suppressed in favour of somnambulism. And yet the way back is never far away and always remains available. We can begin to joyfully create or discover these rituals of re-enchantment; we can begin to feel the deeper sense of belonging at a more visceral level. We are all orphans seeking our way home, finding our way back to our wild forgotten selves, to the ancient drum that beats within all of us – the beat of the Earth, the beat of the Cosmos, calling us back into our kinship with life, into full connection with the Wild Life that we have always been a part of.

I am deeply indebted to the many people who have supported me on this path, and who believed in me and the vision of a gentler world that they too share. I am also so grateful for all of the ways in which Nature has reminded me of the bigger picture, inspired me when I was feeling down, and kept alive my connection when I felt so ostracised by mainstream society. Now it all makes sense, but it has been a long journey of faith and trust.

Stefan Batorijs
Devon, UK
August 2023

A note on language

I have chosen to use the term 'Oriental' within the text as a reference to a body of knowledge and wisdom that arose mostly in China and Japan in antiquity, as opposed to the term East Asian which is a more contemporary format. As an author I am sensitive to the impact of words on others and how certain terms may ostracise some whilst attracting others. I am aware that the term Oriental may appear outdated or part of the colonialisation of language, or how we exoticise non-white cultures, but it is carefully chosen here to describe this body of philosophy as distinct from 'Occidental' culture.

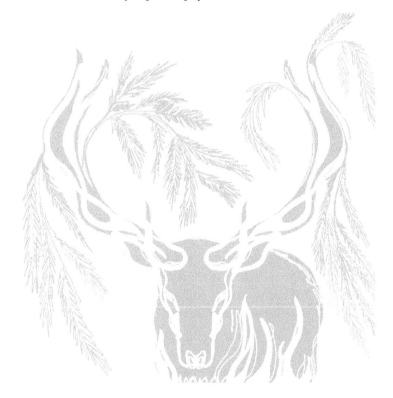

Curlew Dance

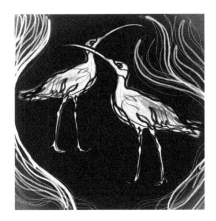

It was that moment in time when dreamy childhood oblivion suddenly gives way to expanding conscious awareness, an individuation process wracked with awareness of separation, awareness of self and other, awareness of sexuality, and awareness of awareness, but mostly a super-awareness of worlds beyond worlds. It is the no-going-back moment of that involuntary step over the threshold of adult imago and into the turbulent and unsheltered waters of existential confusion, ontological searching, and acne.

The date was Easter of 1975, I had just turned 16 and had decided quite uncharacteristically to go and stay with my grandparents in a remote village between the Lake District and the coast, to ostensibly revise for my forthcoming GCE exams. I was a very bright, highly precocious, disruptive pupil who could not take school seriously; my complete lack of respect for authority, plus a distinct failure to see how Jane Austen could remotely relate to my painful teenage angst, and a school run by smelly old sadistic priests was never going to be a good combination for someone who yearned to be out by the riverbank, or making fires away from the bullies. Nevertheless, I persisted with some good chunks of revision until I finally felt the pull of Nature and decided to go for a late-afternoon walk. My favourite walk since childhood was to climb to the top of the 223-metre hill opposite my grandparents' house. The air was cold and refreshing coming in off the Solway Firth, and I felt cleansed and happy as I wandered the lonnin (Cumbrian for lane).

On my way back home, as I was just below the brow of the remote hill, I suddenly stopped and was drawn to an oval-shaped hole in the thick hedge. I crouched down and peered through, and there before me, about 60 feet away, was a group of seven or eight curlews standing in a circle. I cannot even begin to explain what really happened next, because I believe it to be in the realm of the ineffable, a mystic encounter beyond any human language, beyond the comprehension of the analytical reductionist mind.

I have long been hesitant to share this precious, intimate moment with others, for fear that it becomes trivialised, dissected, diluted, or ridiculed, but it is one of the key developmental moments in my life's journey, a definite shift in perception. The reason I share it now is to give a flavour of the type of event that the book is inspired by. These events have powerful totemic and heuristic significance, and occur naturally when we are ready and receptive to such illuminating occurrences. I believe it is of great value to us as Nature therapists that we can be awake and sensitive to these available and revelatory intercessions.

The curlew (*Numenius arquata*, the new moon archer's bow) has always been such an exciting 'wild' bird for me; like the crane of this land. With its tall, upright stance and long, curving bill, it's unmistakeable haunting call is such a joy whenever you hear it, whether on the coast or out on the moors and mires. As I crouched down, silently observing these curlews, something very strange happened. I went into what I can only describe now as a deeply altered state of consciousness; everything fell away from me, it was a complete ego dissolution, I became like vapour, and there was only me (but not me) and the birds up on that bleak hillside. Nothing else existed. My vision shifted; I can't explain, it was sharper, but it was like I saw them, I really saw these exquisite creatures not just as birds to watch, as curlews, but as sentient beings. They appeared larger somehow.

There was no separation between us in the sense that we were ethereal and yet wild, intense beings. It felt almost voyeuristic as I gazed, transfixed, through the gap at their intimate gathering, and at the same time I wondered if they knew I was there. Did they know I was watching? Is it anthropocentric to think that maybe they or something other wanted me to witness this event? Since then, I have had many other similar encounters and experiences that happen spontaneously when out in Nature, and frequently associated with birds.

In their little huddle, they each took it in turns to enter the circle and do what I can only describe as a dance whilst the others watched on; they all did various craning motions and made sounds that seemed to suggest their approval. Sometimes a pair would enter the circle and their dance was an avian tarantella, a mesmerising majestic swirl of wings and necks and beaks; it was a sexual and ancient primal ritual I was witnessing. It reminded me of those elaborate court dances with the very stylised movements, and it occurred to me that maybe the dances were mimicking the birds' display in their coquettish behaviour.

That shift of consciousness created a revelatory perception in me, a 'noetic quality'[1] to my understanding that Nature is paradoxically not there for our edification. These birds were dancing as part of their world, their lives, their social rules and courtship behaviours, regardless of whether a human was there or not. We are not the only ones to inhabit this planet; it is not ours, we share it with other beings who have just as much right to be here as us (and I will return to this theme throughout the book). We don't own this Earth, we don't have this arrogant right to decide how we divide and destroy this place. We are visitors here, and we share our home with other wondrous beings.

I have no idea how much time passed, but it began to turn to dusk, and I wandered back in a trance, no longer the me I was before I went out. I was shocked by what I had seen, like an unexpected gift, struggling to integrate this new revelation into my world. The birds danced for themselves; we are not the centre of everything. Why would they dance if there was nobody there to watch? How did they learn to do those things? My teenage head was confounded and swirling with thoughts. Those birds had shown me beauty and something of pure essence, of Spirit, a glimpse of the True Divine.

Curlew is old French (*cour* + *lieu*) for 'running place'. The collective noun for a gathering of curlews is a *curfew* which means 'to cover the fire', but my fire had in many ways been ignited by these graceful beings. It is also called a salon or a skein, which the Oxford Dictionary describes as 'an element that forms part of a complex or complicated whole: *he weaves together the **skeins** of philosophy, ecology, folklore, and history*'. Maybe that is partly what this book is attempting to do: weave the skeins of life and Nature and healing together, bringing the magic of the curlew dance into another creative form.

This complex, interweaving whole includes us, and I feel it is these kinds of intense experiences which bring us back into unity, and are in fact the web reminding us of why we are here: our purpose is to remember. Our purpose is akin to that of bees – to go out and find the nectar of life and then return to the hive and do our elaborate waggle dance to indicate the path to connection, or the curlew dance, high in the windswept, remote, and undomesticated margins of our psyches.

Strangely, we come across a description of a similar experience from the Nature mystic writer Walter Murray, while visiting a hill geographically very close to my hill, called White Preston:

> the whistle of the curlew is like a silver thread, embroidering a magical pattern across the purple tapestry of moor and fell. Its magic transports me beyond all limitations of time.[2]

Murray also eloquently articulates the feeling of these intense moments of spiritual communion in Nature:

> It sometimes happens, at rare moments in our lives, we are suddenly aware of an altogether new world, different completely from that which we commonly live. We feel as though we stand at the threshold of an undiscovered kingdom; for brief moments we understand life interpreted, we perceive meaning instead of things... I was no longer a single life pushing a difficult way amidst material things, I was part of all creation...it was a baptism into a saner way of living and thinking. It was an outward and visible sign of my inward awareness of at-one-ment.[3]

Are We Suffering?

Many more people are suffering from a form of eco-anxiety about the fate of the Earth, and I sometimes have those desperate feelings of despair, which range from rage to dejection, particularly at the mindless or greedy or fearful felling of trees, and the destruction of the landscape that I have witnessed over the last half a century. However, I do believe that the best antidote for these feelings, which are often characterised by helplessness, is both to protest and to come out to Nature and rejoice in creation and find strength in all that we hold dear, remind ourselves of the daily miracles of life, witness the iridescent beauty all around us, and bring others out to join us.

That's what this book is about: the call to find the places in Nature that we connect with, learn from Mother Nature, and celebrate life; even if (worst-case scenario) we are the orchestra on the *Titanic*, we can hold each other and sing together and know that we did our best.

I'm sure that quite a lot of my sense of outrage comes through in the book, and I thought very carefully about that and whether to keep passion and feelings out of the equation, but eventually I concluded that it was better to be animated and demonstrative than objective and distant.

I was so moved by Greta Thunberg's speech to the World Economic Forum at Davos, Switzerland, in 2019:

> We are now at a time in history where everyone with any insight of the climate crisis that threatens our civilisation – and the entire biosphere – must speak out in clear language, no matter how uncomfortable and unprofitable that may be. We must change almost everything in our current societies. The bigger your carbon footprint is, the bigger your moral duty. The bigger your platform, the bigger your responsibility. Adults keep saying: 'We owe it to the young people to give them hope.' But I don't want your hope. I don't want you to be hopeful. I want you to panic. I want you to feel the fear I feel every day.
>
> And then I want you to act. I want you to act as you would in a crisis. I want you to act as if the house is on fire. Because it is.

If we do care deeply about Nature, we are now frontline, we are vanguards, and sentinels, we are the spokespeople for the dispossessed and the silent voices of the natural world. If Nature can continue to be unconditional, it is a great example for us all. She is doing all she can to rebalance the biosphere, and we can help in the small gestures of our everyday lives. Our spiritual practice of welcoming Nature into our rituals, of aligning with broadly feminine principles, and celebrating the turning of the seasons wherever we are help to grow a coalition of reverent body prayer. There is so much still to be grateful for and so much we can do to build intimacy and regain sensitivity with Nature; not become overwhelmed but take small daily steps towards healing.

The word 'ecotherapy' is made up of two Greek words, *oikos* + *therapeia*. *Oikos* translates as 'home or dwelling', and *therapeia* means 'to look after or take care of'. So ecotherapy then means to take care of our home (in the same way as economy means to 'put our home in order' – literally sort our house out). Thunberg's warning that our house is on fire is particularly apt. Ecotherapy in the purest sense is about recognising our intrinsic dependence on Nature and the Earth as our home and how it's incumbent on us to take care of her. Note that there is nothing in this description which mentions the Earth having to look after us, or about us further exploiting Nature as a resource for therapy.

Obviously, to want to take care of our home, we need to feel again and value that home which requires a significant shift in our cultural perspectives – it's the numbness that allows us to distance ourselves and therefore be complicit in destroying or disregarding our home. It is the predominance of the masculinising of society that has infected us with a set of conditioned values so all-encompassing that we never question that there may be another way – the way of the heart.

By contrast, when we venture tenderly into Nature, we encounter contradictions to that dominant narrative – we encounter death, decay, and impermanence (mindfulness); we encounter the feminine and the archetypes of the sacred feminine, and we have our hearts opened, and our bare souls revealed through an alchemical process (magic); we begin to encounter our own soft inner self that belongs more to the earth and the sky than the illusory comfort of technology.

We soon discover increased sensitivity towards the uniqueness and reality of our place in the Universe, ergo our responsibility; we begin to understand the subtle yet profound interconnections – that nexus of life between all beings, life as one sentient organism, and therefore are compelled to shift our lifestyles and priorities away from the current paradigm of growth, spending, and resource depletion for profit, away from our headlong ecocide, and towards the yearning of the heart.

At its most basic definition, then, ecotherapy posits that in taking care of our home, our household, we extend that care out to all sentient beings, both human and non-human. We broaden our circle of compassion and empathy.

The purest description of therapy is to be kind to someone – to help someone. If you don't feel that you have the capacity to be kind to someone, it may be worth taking time to self-nurture and feel held by Nature before giving to others. I know how it feels when you get burnt out and there's nothing left in the tank; it's time to go out and find the nest of care in the quiet places on the land, to feed directly on pure energy to restore the depleted system – just follow the animals, they know where to go, or learn to dowse these places for your healing.

Therapist John Heron defines 'helping' as supporting and enabling the wellbeing of another person. Can we extend that out to the other-than-human world too? He goes on to say that helping comes from the grace within the human spirit. That grace includes a combination of concern, empathy, prescience, facilitation, and genuineness, or authenticity that is the spiritual heritage of humankind.[4]

Let's now move on to ecopsychology, which has become synonymous with those feelings of grief at the plight of the planet, and remind ourselves of some of the basic premises of that movement. The following are some of ecopsychology's primary principles according to one of its founding fathers, Theodore Roszak:[5]

- There is a synergistic interplay between planetary and personal wellbeing.

- The core of the mind is the ecological unconscious.

- The goal of ecopsychology is to awaken the inherent sense of environmental reciprocity that lies within the ecological unconscious.

- The contents of the ecological unconscious represent the living record of evolution.

- The crucial stage of development is the life of the child.

- The ecological ego matures toward a sense of ethical responsibility with the planet.

- Whatever contributes to small-scale social forms and personal empowerment nourishes the ecological ego.

Please take some time to read these through and see how they feel inside you. The last point speaks directly to the suggestions I'm making about our individual responsibilities for the planet and how we are nurtured within that in our reciprocal relationship as described in the previous points.

If you can hold on to these points as they occur throughout the book, they give an outline and foundation for more elaborate enquiries and explorations alongside Arne Næss's eight-point platform for Deep Ecology. These lists are useful, but, as I said, we have to find our own way, our own truths here. My hope is that within these chapters you may find useful pointers on how to encourage and develop those deeper ecological relationships and not simply regard forest bathing as a bolt-on to your practice, or another exploitation of our precious jewel of life.

If we are suffering, let's give voice to that suffering; let's also create rituals and sacraments of love and joy for the bounteous Earth and re-energise the connection to the seasons, the glory of the wheel turning, the elements, the senses, the simple pleasures and truths of trusting our instinctive selves, finding redemption in all that breathes.

CHAPTER 1

Aesthetic Ecology

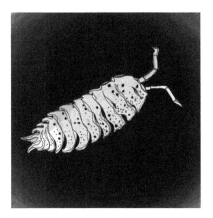

Everybody needs beauty as well as bread, places to play in and pray in,
where nature may heal and give strength to body and soul.

JOHN MUIR[6]

The Human Givens approach is a form of positive psychology that acknowledges the human being as a biological organism with specific emotional needs. One of those givens is attention – to give and receive it is a form of nutrition. I would like to add another emotional need to that list: beauty – to give and receive it is also a form of nutrition.

The beauty of balance

Beauty in Nature and aesthetic ecology is just as important for us as the ecological preservation of individual species or habitats. As John Muir suggests, we need beauty as much as we need bread to live. It's not a romantic ideal; it's essential to our mental wellbeing. Particular places within Nature hold energy – not just visual beauty, but a sense of the vitality and compositional diversity, underground magnetic forces, and other Earth energies detectable by dowsing but felt instinctively through innate or acquired sensitivity. It's vital to protect these places as repositories or sources of Nature's own stores of strength and vitality as energy nodes in the deep subsurface network of energy pathways and mycelium.

Since the 1970s, the UK has experienced a significant biodiversity loss, according to a report prepared for parliament in 2019 called *The State of Nature*.[7] The report describes the UK as 'one of the most nature-depleted countries in the world'. *The State of Nature* report shows that since the 1970s, 41 per cent of all UK species surveyed have declined, while 15 per cent of species within the UK are said to be threatened with extinction; of greatest conservation concern are the UK's priority species, which have declined by 60 per cent.[4]

We need to re-evaluate our conservation and forest management practices to include health and wellbeing as a key factor in how we approach land use, alongside giving greater consideration to the intelligence of Nature, and to establish a code of conduct that recognises the rights of the other-than-human world to be respected as if it was a citizen (e.g., having personhood). Unfortunately, we still take a very objective and detached view on how we manage the land, but the growth of rewilding schemes and the promotion of regenerative agriculture will undoubtedly yield some revelatory findings that support the idea that Nature has the capacity to restore equilibrium by herself, and that equilibrium can be measured by the aesthetic harmony as we perceive it. Key indicator species can take up to 100 years to recolonise a piece of human-disturbed ground, particularly if subject to agricultural run-off and NPK[8] leakage which over-enriches the soil, making it uninhabitable.

The basic rule here is if it looks beautiful to the eye, if it has that aesthetic ecology, then it is probably alright, and doesn't require our intervention.[9] Yes, of course beauty is subjective, but I mean a commonly agreed sense of ecological harmony and balance as felt by the senses. However, beauty or aesthetics are rarely considered within the ecological conversation, either because they are ignored or considered secondary or of inconsequential importance.

To be clear, I am not advocating that we need to objectify Nature for our own amusement, or, as Timothy Morton suggests, put Nature on a pedestal.[10] It comes down to the way that ecological systems harmonise and respond to systemic changes and adaptations. The default position of dynamic balance is continual adjustment around a median evolutionary status, unless we humans introduce changes that overwhelm the system's elastic responsive capabilities.

Ecosystems are strong and yet fragile, responsive, adaptive, and also vulnerable to unencountered alien introductions. Over time, Nature can develop a response which will restore the balance within that system which interacts with and is interdependent on every other adjacent system. We have to trust that that process will yield an outcome that may be at variance with our conservation aims. The recent trend for rewilding has the opportunity to allow this healing to unfold.

When modern destructive grazing animals are excluded, Nature abhors a vacuum, so immediately recolonises itself through a process called Succession Woodland. Areas may start to look scruffy or covered with impenetrable gorse, bracken, and bramble, and other early colonisers, and so people may complain about the wisdom of these changes and the Chaos factor, wanting instead to re-establish order and tradition. These marginal, freshly colonising areas are rich sources of Nature energy or Ki, and are worth exploring on a forest bathing walk or specific intervention. Pioneer species concentrate wild forces and they accumulate towards the ultimate succession.

We could learn so much more and heal more if we can begin to transcend this anthropocentric perspective that puts profit, false security, and a hubristic sense that we are the custodians of Nature and therefore know what's best at the centre of how we operate. Recent discoveries and greater appreciation of ancient indigenous knowledge and custodianship reveal just how little we still know about Nature. For the first time in history, we as a species are responsible for the potential extinction event that will reset Nature on this planet for the next few million years. #naturelivesmatter.

Our interventions need to be considered from a spiritual perspective, a spiritual ecology which includes taking a holistic approach. Nature can look after herself. Our Ecosystems, like Gaia, are always seeking homeostasis. Systems seek balance and continually fine-tune to compensate for dynamic variants within the living system. Issues arise when alien components that have not been a part of the evolution of those ecosystems are suddenly introduced. Much like our own immune systems that respond to viruses and bacteria, if we have not encountered a particular germ, bacteria, virus before, our system has no database for that invasion. Most Westerners have generational genetic memories of TB, polio, cancer, syphilis, and gonorrhoea inside them; these so-called miasms tick away in the background, influencing our evolving immune systems, even though the diseases have been largely eradicated, and now strangely are making a comeback. Forests have immune systems too. A healthy forest can withstand exogenous threats due to the vitality of its components.

Every part of a forest, every tiny plant, moss, lichen, beetle, and fly, has evolved its niche over many millions of years. If we never went near that forest, it would continue to evolve, fine-tune, rebalance and grow. Trees would fall, and other plants would make use of the suddenly available sunlight to expedite growth. The forest canopy forms a shield over the developing nursery of trees below; similarly, the smaller trees, shrubs, and plants at the margin of the forest protect the sides. In a healthy forest that has grown up unmolested, that canopy will have a slight curve to it, so that the winds are channelled over the top and round the sides. When a tree falls over, that space is quickly filled with greenery, a bit like a wound healing; soon the canopy closes in again, and the process continues. This is happening over centuries-long time spans.

If that forest has its natural ecology balanced, and according to various factors like soil type, pH, slope, latitude, and hydrology, it will have a unique and thriving community of plants and creatures, like a green metropolis. The healthy system is full of its vibrant native components; every inch is involved in that constantly evolving process. We may go out to the woods for an hour and conclude that nothing is happening – it is, but it's just not very fast or visible.

Every tiny element of that ecosystem is relevant and vital; every flight of a fly or bee, every bird call, every sighing bough, every fox cough in the night is equally an important part of the matrix of the sentience of this being. The forest resists invasion: each tree can release phytoncides, can concentrate tannins in certain leaves, can shut down in the event of drought, can warn other trees of imminent attack – it's a form of intelligence. (Is it possible that old trees let their neighbours know when they are coming to the end of their lives, so the others can prepare?)

It is generally the species that we have introduced from elsewhere in addition to plant diseases that can have a devastating effect on the forest microbiome. For example, *Rhodedendron ponticum* looks amazing flowering on the slopes of the Himalayas, as it does here too, but it can become invasive – the botanical equivalent of cancer, an energy that is in harmony somewhere else in the Universe, but destructive out of place. *R. ponticum* needs certain key conditions to thrive that mimic its Himalayan origins. Once established, it spreads by increasing its own favourable acidic conditions and nothing much else can grow. A strong robust forest can contain and limit the spread of *R. ponticum* and will not provide the space or optimal conditions for growth. Unfortunately, our temperate rainforests here in the South West and also in many of our upland areas with acidic soils in England, Wales, and Scotland do provide adequately similar conditions to encourage this species that was first introduced by Victorian plant hunters.

In 2020, the outgoing head of the Forestry Commission, Sir Harry Stud-holme suggested that we need to embrace conifers and other exotics as part of our attempts to protect the landscape from a rapidly warming climate and sequester carbon for the future. I think that we are going to need all the non-invasive, non-intrusive alien trees we can hang on to. Introduced trees that have seamlessly integrated into the landscape are likely to provide a biodiversity that will be useful over the next half a century. Trees like sweet chestnut, London plane, Douglas fir, some cherry species, and eucalyptus all have a contribution to make to our bastard landscape and should not be treated as unwanted migrants. Let's embrace the biodiversity and the variety that these plants bring us. We are no longer in the luxurious position to cultivate an entire Nature reserve for a single dwindling species of butterfly.

The fundamental importance of beauty

Beauty has an inherent value of its own. This has been recognised throughout the ages, going back beyond Plato and other early Greek philosophers, who debated whether beauty was objective or subjective, and whether it was part of the virtues that were held in esteem. In the *Symposium,* Plato discusses his theory of forms, stating that the manifest beauty we witness is a material form of the eternal and intelligible beauty which is invisible.

My experience of beauty in Nature is more than just 'eye pastures', more than just a temporary fix of mind tranquilliser – it is a sense of the Divine made manifest in form and the perfection of the dynamic intelligence of Nature. All landscapes within the UK have been manipulated by man, including the National Park that I live in here on Dartmoor, a 954 km² area of predominantly granite upland and a stunning, wild, moody place of moors and steep valleys. Dartmoor attracts about 3 million visitors a year, and I would suggest that it is the wild expanses and the 'wild' Dartmoor ponies that form the major attraction of this place. It is the subconscious desire for wildness that attracts, as it speaks to this 'archaic' (Jung's term) part of our psyche. And yet Dartmoor is entirely artificial – it is one of our earliest ecological catastrophes.

Early tribes found a place with dense tree cover and a much warmer climate than today that was the perfect place for settlements, with some commanding views and rich resources. Over time, the stripping back of the tree cover led to serious soil erosion, exposing the bedrock, which resulted in the decimation of the ecology and negatively impacted the local microclimate. Dartmoor became barren and the tribes deserted for pastures new. What remains is a monoculture of coarse grasses and peat bogs which have acidified the landscape, catchments, and rivers.

Nature can very quickly repair this damage and reverse it, and when one wanders around the moor, there are several places where grazing has been limited and the wound-healing, reforesting, succession woodland process is in full flow. It is the grazing of cattle, sheep, ponies, and deer that arrests this recovering capacity of the land. Excluding livestock would radically change the shape and contents of the landscape and lead to the growth of a new primary forest, in turn favourably impacting the microclimate. An older hierarchy of forest dwellers, reintroduced with great care, would lead to a new but vibrant landscape where humans could benefit as much as animals, trees, and soil. I'm not advocating wolves, but other management species and predators could restore balance and vitality.

Much of Dartmoor is called forest, and yet there are few trees there. Even our three last remaining isolated pockets of old woods, our northern temperate rainforests such as Wistman's Wood, are struggling to maintain their ecologies due to the ravages of grazing, weather, soil pH, and biodiversity loss. If these areas were fenced off from everything including humans and rabbits, reseeded and replanted, and a natural windbreak created for some of the more fragile species to gain a foothold, in 10–20 years we would see a remarkable transformation and another version of beauty to behold.[11]

We find beauty in these remote and isolated places as they bring our minds to rest, they remind us of our genetic and psychic ancestry, and they captivate our hearts and imaginations. We seem to need to seek out direct contact and communion with life in its raw, wild essence. Nan Shepherd, the Cairngorm explorer and writer, says, 'beauty is not adventitious but essential', which reinforces the idea of beauty as soul food, as an elixir for health.

Interestingly, simply looking at images of wilderness will also produce a de-stressing, 'horizoning' effect, expansive and indeterminate, reassuring, yet also in some way unsettling, as it distracts us from our condensed constellations of immediate concerns. Dr Miyazaki's work of exposing people to images of the forest within clinical settings demonstrated what Roger Ulrich had first identified back in 1984: looking at Nature either on a screen or through a hospital window led to reduced healing times and fewer complications post-surgery.[12] Miyazaki's experiment demonstrated that viewing pictures of trees for 90 seconds had beneficial effects on the nervous system, and led to sensations of being 'comfortable', 'relaxed', and 'natural'. Images of the city were used as controls.[13]

These clinical research results help to support the concept that Nature enhances physiological and psychological wellbeing, as well as benefitting cognitive function, reducing heart rate, and lowering stress levels. Biophilic responses are hardwired into the brain, and exposure to Nature plays a key role in self-perception and spiritual wellbeing.

However, looking at beauty is a passive experience and very different from the immersive experience of being surrounded by beauty – being inside the forest, bathing in a mountain stream, or sitting silently and contemplating Nature all around us. A 2D image avoids the wildness and the life breath of Nature, and the exposure to unpredictability which I believe we need in our lives – it's a muscle that needs flexing within us: the underlying Palaeolithic self needs stimulation and edginess. People who don't have access to the natural environment can achieve benefits from watching nature videos, and technology is currently being developed to utilise virtual reality headsets for an immersive nature experience.[14]

Wabi sabi

The Japanese have this wonderful term *wabi sabi* for the experience of the simplicity and rawness or roughness of Nature, that is summed up perfectly by this concept of finding truth and strength within Nature and immersion in the natural world.

Wabi sabi refers to a philosophical principle related to Buddhist values. Meditating on the landscape to understand that beauty is transient, impermanent, imperfect, and incomplete or empty, we find sanctuary in the open, empty isolation of Nature. Much like the Dartmoor landscapes which evoke a lonely, serene, melancholic feeling, especially with a cold wind blowing (which is virtually always). Much loved by Taoists too, other characteristics of *wabi sabi* include asymmetry, austerity, imperfections, modesty, intimacy, and the appreciation of the transience of everything relating to the forces of nature and natural objects.

Komorebi

Another related though less desolate Japanese term has no direct translation, but refers somewhat romantically to the experience of sunlight filtering through the branches of trees, best experienced early in the morning or at dusk. *Komorebi* refers to how the beauty of this moment fills us with positive energy and a good heart. I become absolutely mesmerised by the patterns sunlight makes dancing on the leaves of the forest floor, and the shadow shapes in negative spaces. *Komorebi* reminds us to stop and take in these moments of beauty and peace. The very fact that the Japanese have a word for this in their language says so much about their culture. I invite my students to contemplate this delicate play of light in the Devon woods, especially after the rain.

Patterns in Nature

Nature has the capacity to display its infinite design within the immediate moment and the observable world. Every aspect of Nature, large and small, shares a mathematical signature with every other component, both singularly different and simultaneously connected, individual and composite all at once. Patterns in Nature can be witnessed empirically, and from these observations subjective deductions can be formed which speak to our spiritual understanding as an aspect of being, not belief. Just a reminder, we are spiritual entities attempting physical experience, and evidence for the Divine signature provides comfort, familiarity, and connection.

This is a participatory Universe, and we are all complicit players and components in this meta-conscious mystery play, we are vital and valued collaborators. There is no separation between the manifestation of phenomena and us as the observers of these processes; we are all somehow aspects of this metaphysical Russian doll. Artists deploy observation and imagination as they witness the beauty in the natural world; their observation processes are more intuitive than perhaps a scientific study, their methods and concerns at variance with each other, so two people may observe the same phenomena but record them differently.

In order to fully understand Nature, including its expression of beauty, we need to allow ourselves to become receptive to the beauty that lies within us. To fully integrate our knowledge of Nature calls for us to discover those aspects within us; the beauty we observe and are attracted to is purely a reflection of the beauty that exists within us, and our innate response to beauty can say much about how we relate to our inner life and heart. The environmental scientist and activist Rachel Carson encapsulated this sentiment about beauty in her speech:

I believe natural beauty has a necessary place in the spiritual development of any individual or any society. I believe that whenever we destroy beauty, or whenever we substitute something man-made and artificial for a natural feature of the earth, we have retarded some part of man's spiritual growth.[15]

Adopting a purely scientific approach to Nature requires us to deny or suppress that spiritual relationship, that intimate conversation, and conversely opening ourselves up to our feelings and intuition makes us receptive to deep insights that can nourish and nurture our personal development and spiritual journeys. The poet and visionary William Blake opined that 'The tree which moves some to tears of joy is in the eyes of others only a green thing which stands in the way... As a man is, so he sees.'[16] I would also add that as a man sees, so he is; when we filter our experiences of Nature, we inure ourselves to the sacrality and beauty we behold in order to carry out immoral acts of destruction and scientific vandalism, and become further armoured against the nutrition of beauty, and our souls wither and dry up inside us in a barren prison of objectivity and rational superiority.

Fractals and spirals are encoded reminders of the deeper mathematical harmony within the Universe, existing long before we emerged from the swamp. Fractals are beautiful, self-replicating shapes visible in the veins in our bodies and mirrored in the lightning in the sky. They are hypnotic geometrical forms made up of smaller and smaller versions of themselves, as can be seen in fern fronds and river estuaries viewed from space.

The arcs of spirals can be described by the Golden Mean (or Golden Ratio) and the Fibonacci series of numbers, visible in the double-helix shapes of sunflower seed heads and certain cacti leaves, and encoded into the sacred architecture of Chartres Cathedral. Fractals and spirals come together in romanesco broccoli, with their amazing mini spirals forming bigger spirals.

As an experiment, I invite you to go out and spend some time seeking spirals and fractals within Nature, and observe the effect on your person. How does the discovery of these interrelated forms impact your consciousness, and how do you locate these forms and the flow they imply within you? The DNA helix is an obvious example at a very literal level, but what else can you sense when you encounter the simple and exquisite beauty within the pragmatic development of phenomena? Does blood flow in a spiral?

Bringing fractals and spiral shapes into awareness with participants can be a rewarding activity, whether we can observe fractals within the patterns of branch development in a tree silhouetted against a sky, or spirals within the tactile form of a shell, an acorn cup, or the underside of a fir cone. The satisfying beauty within the visual component connects powerfully when we have that tactile investigation to bring the physicality and dimensionality into play. Both energetic forms are manifest at scale from microcosm up to cosmic or galactic forms; a recent study attempted to find corollaries between the structure of the brain and the structure of galaxies, and found some interesting similarities or parallels in how they functioned as expressions of intelligence at differing scales.[17] Even the Earth orbits in a spiral as it glides through the darkness.

Divine beauty

Beauty and intelligence abound within the Universe, and aesthetic considerations are implied within our practices as Forest Medicine practitioners; ignoring the intelligence within the beauty reduces our work to nothing more than another consumer experience with a time limit and a consciousness separation. Engaging with this cosmic expression of consciousness and its invitation to participate realigns us back to Nature, and gives us an increased sense of vitality and health.

John O'Donohue, the wonderful and sadly missed Irish poet, theologian, and philosopher, wrote *Divine Beauty: The Invisible Embrace* in 2004. I cannot compete with his heavenly lyrical eloquence and profound insights, so I point the reader towards his book, as he elevates the idea of beauty to another level, no longer a superficial aesthetic but a calling to our souls. In one of his final interviews, he shared this feeling that beauty was more about rounded, substantial becoming than it was about nice loveliness. O'Donohue regarded beauty as a kind of homecoming, offering us a greater sense of grace and elegance, depth and fullness to our lives.

O'Donohue also wrote about how the human soul is hungry for beauty, which leads me to think about the people who never get to experience beauty in their lives, how depleted they may feel, or empty and unfulfilled. Finding beauty in even the smallest flower or patch of weeds or the colours of the sunset can be such a strong tonic for the soul. It is clear to me that we need to place more effort in supporting people from inner-city areas with low incomes or limited opportunities to have the chance to escape into Nature and have an immersion in beauty, a Nature beauty bath, as well as bringing more Nature to cities where its amelioratory effect can be measured in health terms.

The Deep Ecology movement created by Arne Næss in Norway started with the premise of an aesthetic approach to ecology and valuing beauty as one aspect of the inherent value of Nature. Point 1 of the Deep Ecology

8-point platform, a kind of manifesto for universal principles and values, declares that the 'flourishing of human and non-human life on Earth have value in themselves. These values are independent of the usefulness of the non-human world for human purposes.'[18]

This point also reflects a further distinction of the Deep Ecology movement in a belief that when non-human beings experience joy, then we experience joy too. Joy and beauty are intrinsically linked and have a value beyond their appropriation for advertising imagery. Beauty is so often associated with glossy images of youth in an attempt to sell us the latest 'beauty' product aimed at making us immortally young, but true beauty belongs to us all and is transient. Beauty is a feeling, not a condition that can be commodified, and discovering the beauty of Nature can be revelatory and deeply therapeutic in its effect.

The German geologist, poet, and writer Hans Cloos sums it up by writing:

> Why does man find beauty in a landscape? Is it not because he is a part of nature, inwardly subject to nature's laws, because he has an unconscious insight into the internal order of the earth, into the rhythm of its repetitions, the harmony of its lines and surfaces and the balanced interplay of its parts? And does not our delight in the contemplation of nature grow out of the harmony between the music of our own soul and the music of the earth?[19]

Consciousness

Although not from a scientific background but from a practical outdoor one, there is always a part of me that needs one of two things or even both in order to fully trust something: I need some hard irrefutable evidence coming from a reliable source (without vested interests in skewing facts in a particular way) or the somatic experiencing and knowing of my body, and for that to hold true over successive encounters. Being a skeptical (but not cynical), pragmatic person, I have also been at times the doubting Thomas, needing to touch the wound in order to believe.

I don't just take everything on faith, or superstition, but look for what rings true for me deep down in the core of my intuitive knowing, and to then robustly challenge that knowing and look for a more objective enquiry into the ontology and epistemology of the phenomena encountered. I have had many 'spiritual' or mystical experiences in Nature that seem to defy rational thought, science, and objective reality, events that have taken me far beyond the daily limits of my reasoning mind and restricted consciousness into realms of the unseen worlds that permeate our waking ordinary realities. The American psychologist and mystic writer William James offers this insight which also points towards the ephemerality of these states:

> Our normal waking consciousness, rational consciousness as we call it, is but one special type of consciousness, whilst all about it, parted from it by the filmiest of screens, there lie potential forms of consciousness entirely different. We may go through life without suspecting their existence; but apply the requisite stimulus, and at a touch they are there in all their completeness, definite types of mentality which probably somewhere have their field of application and adaptation. No account of the universe in its totality can be final which leaves these other forms of consciousness quite disregarded. How to regard them is the question – for they are so discontinuous with ordinary consciousness. Yet they may determine attitudes though they cannot furnish

formulas, and open a region though they fail to give a map. At any rate, they forbid a premature closing of our accounts with reality.[20]

As a student of the edges of consciousness and the transpersonal, this notion of going beyond the perceived limits of the human body or mind has been brought into sharp experiential focus by my spontaneous involuntary excursions into mystical states in Nature. These glimpses into other realms, into Aldous Huxley's 'Mysterium tremendum', feel strangely purposeful and full of portent, though that could just be my ego trying to re-establish some control over affairs. They share many of the qualities and epiphanies of psychedelic states and transcendent experiences. Renowned Neuroscientist Iain McGilchrist describes consciousness as being 'ontologically primitive' – the primary and fundamental reality of the cosmos. This is particularly evident when we attune within natural settings to the rhythm of Nature.

I have a very strong sense that there is so much more to know and understand about Nature, about matter, energy, and consciousness, so many hidden realms invisible to the naked eye existing within our own, and to which we also belong and are connected, interpenetrating, flowing, communicating between us.

Shinrin-yoku has become popular and gained credibility from its inception in Japan partly due to the development of the portable measuring equipment that can make accurate analyses of participants' blood, saliva, and heart rate in the forest. This medical science is undoubtedly important and serves to confirm what we may have intuitively known all along: that being in Nature is largely good for our wellbeing. I must caution against getting overly transfixed by the medical results and the implications of these studies, valuable as they are in understanding exactly what is happening; sometimes our obsession with the stats can blind us to the trees burning all around us.

These other realms of consciousness or intelligence are present and can intersect our lives at the subtlest of levels, each realm a delicate permeable barrier, a spiritual osmotic gradient. Information flows in both directions and then occasionally we slip through into another place and return different. These times/places where the 'veil lies thinnest' have been alluded to by mystics and neophytes alike over the centuries, and are very familiar and well understood places within indigenous shamanic traditions from around the world. One of the themes of this work is to explore how we can access our own conscious states within a Nature setting, and the context of those revelatory intense experiences, how they sit within our own cultural reference points: positive or negative perceptions and biases, our carefully constructed but limited versions of reality.

In his new book *The Matter with Things* (2023), McGilchrist describes how we have developed a reductionist materialistic viewpoint, due to left-brain dominance, and by contrast how we need to see the bigger picture, taking a more holistic and embodied perspective, and allowing our imagination and intuition to flourish in order to properly tune in to what is real in the Cosmos.

These glimpses of other textures of reality can open psychic doors, or they can help to find closure on old wounds and soul business stuff. In all cases, these deeper moments of lucidity belong to us, as we belong to them: are we in fact comprised of more consciousness than material being, or is consciousness rooted in our biology? Random superconscious events form part of our belonging within the pantheon of Nature, and part of our evolutionary heritage or phylogenesis as animals, as species amongst species, not the hegemony of the human mind.

The invitation for full sensory engagement in forest bathing is both universal and culturally sensitive, particularly our specific social relationships to Nature, and the stories we tell ourselves and our children. Everything alive has intelligence, everything is both expression of and participant in universal consciousness – the one-song which is embodied, not a separate, isolated, individualised exceptionalism. Consciousness arises from our feelings within the body, the aggregation of bodily intelligence – the messages we receive from the sensory and nervous systems, in this respect consciousness is, 'a global function that emerges from but extends beyond our immediate anatomy'.[21]

Our consciousness is the means by which we apprehend the phenomena of life and a complex universe, both the inner and outer, it is the lens through which we perceive and interpret reality, but also the means to transcend it. Downregulating the mind and listening to and with the body through forest bathing practices offers us both a stronger sense of 'self' and a closer appreciation of the mystery of belonging in a vast bewildering Cosmos.

CHAPTER 2

The Universe of Nature and the Nature of the Universe

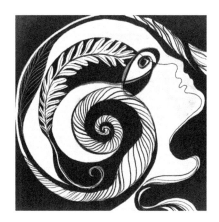

Everyone who is seriously involved in the pursuit of science becomes convinced that a spirit is manifest in the laws of the Universe – a spirit vastly superior to that of man, and one in the face of which we with our modest powers must feel humble.

ALBERT EINSTEIN[22]

Origin of the Universe

Why delve into the origin of the Universe in a book about forest bathing? Well, I think it's important to have a sense of scale and context in our enquiries and pursuits, and as I discuss later, if we can arrive at a commonly agreed evolutionary origin of life, we can then process forward into contentious esoteric or metaphysical topics together, celebrating our common kinship with all things, which can then inform our position relative to the forests that we immerse ourselves in. It's foundational and respectful.

Evolution is the story of the great unfolding that has led us to where we are now. The Scottish-American conservationist and mountaineer John Muir once remarked that 'The clearest way into the Universe is through a forest wilderness', as he quite rightly found all the elements of evolution right there.

There are currently a number of competing theories about the origin of the Universe, including but not limited to the following:

- The Universe has always existed (steady state) in some form and is eternal.

- There was another Universe before ours.

- Ours is just one of many possible 'multiverses'.

- The Creationist or theistic evolution theory, which holds that an omnipresent god or deity created the Universe and all the physical and biological processes that exist.

The current prevailing scientific theory is that the Universe as we know it began with the 'Big Bang' event around 13.8 billion years ago. The universe was created *ex nihilo* – literally from nothing. All of the energy that exists in the entire Universe was held in a single infinitesimal point, a *singularity* smaller than an atom which exploded with unimaginable force. Within those first moments, subatomic nuclei were formed. Within the first 380,000 years, the primordial particles of life were formed into the atoms which would lead to the creation of galaxies and stars, and ultimately you and I.

Do we ever actually cease to exist in some form or other? Do the elemental particles that made us just get recycled into something else for ever and ever? Entropy comes into play here, of course.

The shockwaves from that initial primordial event are still expanding out into space and can be measured. There is a wonderful, enhanced photograph taken by the European Space Agency's Planck space telescope in 2013 of this residual cosmic microwave background radiation.[23] This radiation allows us to measure the existence and timing of the Big Bang, and the expansion of space relative to our position in it. The Universe is expanding, and that means space-time is expanding, and the expansion is accelerating. The Universe is alive; it has a finite beginning and will have a finite end.

Many astrophysicists and cosmologists have described the unfolding development of the Universe in terms such as 'intelligent', 'sentient', and 'elegant'. Such anthropomorphic terms are rarely associated with scientists, especially Prof Brian Cox who prefers to describe this 'feeling of elation when something about Nature is understood and seen to be elegant'.[24] Brian Swimme and Thomas Berry in their excellent book on this topic, *The Universe Story*, describe the Universe as 'a coherent whole, a seamless multilevelled creative event. The graceful expansion of the original body is the life blood of all future bodies in the Universe'.[25] Compare this statement with the classical Taoist text *The Tao Te Ching*, which states that 'non-existence is the antecedent of Heaven and Earth, and existence is the Mother of the myriad things'.

There is a hint in Cox's quote of an organising principle in Nature, and when we roam around in Nature and encounter evidence of this cosmic order, whether it's a fractal pattern in a fern, a murmuration of starlings, the V formation of geese flying overhead, or the divine signature of spirals (Fibonacci sequence), we are captivated like children again, instantly lifted, and filled with a sense of awe, of comfort, and of satisfaction perhaps. I believe this recognition of form and of pragmatic, unembellished beauty constitutes a large part of what heals us in Nature. It reminds us (with a reassuring familiarity that bypasses the intellect) of this sense of belonging mixed with deep, immersive fascination, as in my 16-year-old self's encounter with the curlews. All mundane worries and tribulations are dissolved in the embrace of the Cosmos.

This intimation of what Swimme and Berry term an 'originating power', a grand design, or an intelligence playing out across our lives is, I believe, an immeasurable component of restoration and amelioration in Nature – direct access to the source. This is not simply an excuse for the growth of formal religion or the need for belief systems that reflect a defect or weakness in our psyche, a need for superstition, or to attribute meaning to a monotheistic god or a formal structure of reason, purpose, or fear. This is about recognising the panpsychism of the Universe: all matter, all life is ultimately connected through an infinite matrix of sentience, and the signs and characteristics of that process are all around us (and within us) if we care to look in the right places. When we momentarily step aside from our frenetic, desperate, sometimes neurotic lives, and instead just sit ourselves down in a wood or meadow, or by a stream, we instantly dial into that unbroken and ineffable web of belonging. This must surely be our motivation for leading others out of buildings and back into the natural world of diversity and abundance.

Contemporary physics has demonstrated that nothing in the Universe exists in isolation, and we are now discovering the subtle ways in which everything is dependent for its existence in relation to everything else. Is the Universe self-aware?

That colossus of cosmology Stephen Hawking considered himself an atheist and did not believe in God, yet he acknowledged the 'fine-tuning' process that led to the creation of life was problematic from a physics perspective. This leads us to the Anthropic Cosmological Principle or Fine-tuning.

Sir Fred Hoyle, a very eminent Cambridge Astro-physicist in the 1950s, stated that:

> If you wanted to produce carbon and oxygen in roughly equal quantities by stellar nucleosynthesis, there are two levels you have to fix, and your fixing would have to be just where these levels are actually found to be. Another put-up job? ... I am inclined to think so. A common sense interpretation of the facts suggests that a superintellect has monkeyed with physics, as well as with chemistry and biology, and that there are no blind forces worth speaking about in nature.[26]

Fine-tuning

When one studies the complexity, 'randomness', and simplicity of the great unfolding cosmic interactions at the very beginning of the Universe, one is struck by the multiple ways in which everything could have turned out so differently. The early primordial formation of the two building blocks of life, hydrogen and helium, seemed chaotic and haphazard, and yet led inexorably towards the evolution of life as we know it, and what we term the laws of Nature.

One of the mysteries of creation is that scientists can see that there was a perfect balance between matter and antimatter, and then at some point, a few minute elementary particles known as baryons (numbering roughly 1 in 30 million particles) tilted it towards matter, of which the Universe is largely composed; this is known as baryonic asymmetry. Similarly, the Universe somehow did not collapse back into a black hole at the Big Bang event (but perhaps that had been the outcome many millions of times before).

The forces required to seed the atoms that led to the gas clouds were quite precise and finite. If the spatial and gravitational forces had been slightly weaker, stars would not have exploded into the supernovae that seeded the elements for growth throughout the Universe. Had the Universe established a stronger gravitational force, all the stars would have exploded in a very brief time, rather than the billions of years required for the development of life to unfold. This is the 'fine-tuning' of the natural laws that emerged at the beginning of time, and reflects the integral nature and organising purpose behind this elegant process.

Another significant aspect of this fine-tuning concept is the creation of the Earth, and the conditions necessary for the creation of life. It is difficult to imagine how the same set of circumstances that led to the formation of the Earth could ever exist in any other part of the Universe. The size, formation, composition, position, association, temperature, orbital ellipse and tilted spin axis, influence of the moon and the outer planets; all the twists and turns of how the Solar System gravitationally formed and influenced our position relative to the Sun are so complex and infinitely random, it is a miracle that we are here.

Another British Astrophysicist, George Ellis, summarises this idea: 'Amazing fine-tuning occurs in the laws that make this [complexity] possible. Realisation of the complexity of what is accomplished makes it very difficult not to use the word "miraculous" without taking a stand as to the ontological status of the word.'[27]

According to the Drake equation, a speculative estimate of the chances of the existence of another planet capable of supporting complex extraterrestrial life is about 1 in 60 billion. It is outside the focus of this book to explore the convoluted and chance events that led to our current status, but there is an accumulative effect of the increase of chance with every evolutionary event within the fine-tuning. The 'Rare Earth Hypothesis' argues that the origin of life on Earth and the development of biological complexity requires an improbable combination of astrophysical and geological conditions and chance events.[28]

Cox states that:

There are a vast number of chance events in our past that could have happened differently, and changing any one of them would have meant that we wouldn't be here...our existence is far too contingent on a series of chance events stretching back to the formation of the Solar System and beyond.[29]

Cox asks us whether we should feel irrelevant or valuable when we contemplate our lives and how lucky we are to be here, but I think again we can return to this idea that we are simply fragments or fractals of super-consciousness expressing itself through patterns, forms and self-awareness. Swimme and Berry state:

> Each region of the Universe then and now is permeated with self-organising dynamics in latent form. These ordering patterns hide until the material structures and free energy of the region reach that particular complexity and intensity capable of drawing such patterns forth.[30]

The debate over whether events in the Universe happen by chance or by order has been raging within philosophers' and physicists' circles for hundreds of years, and French writer Voltaire famously declared, 'Chance is a word devoid of sense, nothing can exist without a cause.'

Let's return to Swimme and Berry's earlier statement that the Universe is 'a coherent whole' and a 'seamless, multilevelled creative event'. This is exactly, directly what we access when we step into the wild, or gaze up at the stars. They go on to state, 'The graceful expansion of the original body is the life blood of all future bodies in the Universe.' I interpret that in this context as meaning that the 'Originating Power' gracefully expanded itself to seed life everywhere. What also then follows from this statement is the assertion that the original body is the life blood of all future bodies, so that every aspect of creation has inherently encoded within it some cosmic DNA of the 'Originating Power'.

If we look around us, the evidence of that is everywhere. Not only the key elements that are the building blocks of life such as hydrogen, iron, carbon, and oxygen, but how the four fundamental laws of Nature that serve to organise everything are acting upon every particle of the Universe, so that there is a direct connection between a sycamore seed spiralling down to the ground and the formation of galaxies and stars. These four laws of Nature are gravity, electromagnetism, strong nuclear force, and weak nuclear force. They became separate but they emanated from the One; although described as separate, they act in unity, each being in continuous relationship with the others as representations of that original cosmogenesis, and, of course, all acting on us and through us, in every moment of our lives.

Our selves in Nature

What has all this got to do with Nature therapy? The point is, once we can achieve some consensus about the singularity event, this unique point of origination, we can then move forward together and explore further into the reaches of uncertainty and increasing subjectivity, having established our mutually agreed foundation. This argument is particularly anchoring when dealing with sceptics and cynics. We may have completely distinct or mutually exclusive trajectories, values and beliefs, but if we can agree on the science or genesis of our common ground, we can explore these eco-mysteries together.

Now we are on a shared journey with a shared ancestry, and may discover a common purpose. Contrast this with many artificial therapeutic and psychosocial relationships where we are seen as being in some way separate and distinct from our clients. We are seen as the arbiters of growth, holders of power, and dispensers of goodness and knowledge rather than collaborators in our quest for wholeness. We often talk of 'holding space' for a client, but space is holding us as one indivisible being.

Everything that we are dealing with now had an origin in the primordial past. Out in Nature, we are so much more acutely aware of this interplay of all elements. The four synchronous laws of Nature are acting upon us directly but outside of our awareness, and if we know where to look, they manifest before us. At any time, being in Nature is an invitation to consider our organicity, our smallness, our uniqueness, our animal selves, our quantum selves, and our forest antecedent selves.

I believe it also starts to dissolve or annihilate the ego sense of separateness and distinctness, in contrast to being in the counsellor's office, which can reinforce a sense of segregation and enclosure. When I'm out in the woods with a client, I'm acutely aware that the whole alive forest, the trees, plants, birds, insects, creatures are conscious of our presence, leaning in to hear; they too are part of the continuum, may contribute to our wellbeing, and we are their brethren, their kinfolk. There is an irresistible interpenetration of beingness. We don't need to take everything too seriously either!

If we take these arguments too far, we are in danger of falling into 'anthropo-narcissism', the belief that we are the centre of all that exists, and that all matter is here to affirm our existence or our personal divinity, or variations of the notion that if we are part of Nature, then all our actions are natural and therefore valid. We are distinctly unpredictable animals with a will and a consciousness, which means we sometimes act in ways that aren't in alignment with our organic continuum and the values and virtues associated with the natural world as described by Taoists, Greek philosophers, and mystics alike (and who we will come on to later).

This unbroken evolutionary process that proceeds from the Big Bang leads us inevitably towards an appreciation that our bodies and the rare trace elements that we contain can only be forged in the immense heat and pressure of an exploding star – a supernova. To paraphrase Carl Sagan and Moby, we are indeed all made of stars.[31] The iron inside us that we need to remain healthy is the same iron in the Earth's crust and core, the same iron that came from the exploding furnace of the stars.

This is not meant to sound overly dramatic, but to convey the notion that when we are outside working with someone, we are not separate and distinct entities but continuous expressions of consciousness in relative amounts of materiality and solidity. We can look up at the sky, or look down into the soil, relaxing the ego, coming to know that we are a part of this infinite dance of supreme consciousness called Universe, and that this other person/animal/plant is too; we are all seeking the most fundamentally successful ways to express ourselves, a balance of self and soul purpose perhaps.

A critical or deeper ontological enquiry may seem over-elaborate or subordinate to the task at hand, but by holding within us the notion of our place in the stars whilst we are out amongst the trees – themselves part of some deep cosmic tryst – we can reflect on our therapeutic journeys within a grounded expansive context, even with all our own personal, religious, and sociopolitical perspectives. In Nature, our wild selves revert seamlessly back to our place within the Universe, the Unity-verse. Although meditation points in that same direction, forest bathing embraces our physicality, sensuality, and temporality as an antidote to our perception of plurality, the fear of our mortality, and the chains that bind our love. Stepping out under the stars, our hopes, grief, and cares can be seen from an understanding of our 'immanence', our place within the Universe. Researchers are desperate to quantify this 'awe' effect and define its parameters.

The debate over the origin of the Universe is one of those rare discussions where science, philosophy, and theology intersect. Some scientists are happy to acknowledge that questions like 'What existed before the Universe created space-time?' and 'Why is the Universe here?' are beyond human comprehension; they are transcendent realities and mysteries of the ineffable. Albert Einstein said in his early life that he wanted to ask God *how* the Universe began, but as he got older, he only wanted to ask God *why* the Universe *had* begun.

We must look big, outwards to the galaxies, and we must look small, inwardly to molecules, atoms, and quantum particles to discover the patterns of intelligence within Nature. That is ultimately what science is all about, or as Professor Cox describes it, 'about shapes and patterns in Nature and what they reveal about the way in which the Universe works'.[32] We are Universe, so it is good to delve deep into our origins and our composition to understand our behaviours and pathologies.

Einstein said:

> A human being is a part of the whole called by us the 'Universe', a part limited in time and space. He experiences himself, his thoughts and feeling as something separated from the rest, a kind of optical delusion of his consciousness. This delusion is a kind of prison for us, restricting us to our personal desires and to affection for a few persons nearest to us. Our task must be to free ourselves from this prison by widening our circle of compassion to embrace all living creatures and the whole of nature in its beauty.[33]

Even if (like me) you are not a professional physicist, I'm sure you can begin to see how invaluable it is to get a sense of our connection, our unity, our UNI-verse as Einstein says, as opposed to our duality, our separation, or delusion of separation in the Cartesian sense. Healing of the psyche proportionally arises from the acceptance of these fundamental laws of Nature, rather than the enticing but vacuous social media-proliferated view of virtual immortality.

We are our own avatars. The Universe is perfectly imperfect, and so are we. If we place our faith in Nature, we align ourselves with Beauty and Love, or at the very least we can come to respect all the infinite expressions of Nature of which we are a part, of that vast continuum of cosmic expression, from spiral galaxies right down to the micro-organisms that have made their homes in some of the most inhospitable environments on the planet, including our guts. (Micro-organisms that preceded us, and that converted the atmosphere from anaerobic to aerobic, permitting the growth of more complex life-forms, and which will probably be here long after we are gone – so much for intelligence!)

Having cast a cursory glance over the Cosmic or transcendental origin of the Universe from a scientific perspective, it feels wholly appropriate to turn our attentions to how philosophy emerged from these fundamental questions about life, the Universe, and everything. We will begin with the origin of philosophy in the West and the foundation of the first school of philosophy, and find links with Eastern ideas from around the same time.

Beauty and the Bullfinch

It's a mild early January morning as I sit down to write; the frantic hiatus of the festive season has deflated and given way to the dull, muted tones of winter under a claustrophobic blanket of stratus cloud. The air is still and silent, and searching for inspiration, I gaze dreamily out into my back garden. Suddenly, there are two pairs of bullfinches sitting in the hedge ten feet away. Wow! I am instantly stunned by the shockingly vivid colours of their plumage, made all the more vibrant and psychedelic in contrast with the drab browns and greys of the bare winter backdrop.

I'm just completely mesmerised by the beauty of these beings: the males have this almost indescribable iridescent pink-reddish-orange chest, a harlot's lipstick, a colour to lose yourself in. The Latin name for this bird is *Pyrrhula pyrrhula* from ancient Greek meaning 'flame-coloured' – twice! This is further highlighted by the soft, warm blue-grey back, white stripes, and sooty black head. You could live in a house of these colours or you could understand how fashion ever got started with these outrageous bright, coquettish displays, and how early humans may have adorned themselves to mimic these magnificent colourful birds. You expect to see these colours in a tropical rainforest, and they seem somehow disproportionally bright in the monotone Devon winter.

I am always captivated by bird visitors to my small backyard; even the humble yet proud robin and the noisy, garrulous house sparrows have me entranced with their social gangs, and I feel very privileged to host such exotic birds as the bullfinches in winter (one year a blackcap took up winter residence here instead of migrating, and sang all night, every night!). These welcome guests remind me of the beauty of life, distract me from my tasks, and I marvel at perfect wildness so close to home. I have always had a deep affinity with birds since I was a child, and they have been associated with most of my 'spiritual' experiences as I describe in the book.

The bullfinch episode serves as a good example of how Nature can elevate us beyond mundanity, lead us back to a place where just for a fleeting moment all that exists is just us and this other exotic wild being somehow in communion with us. It pulls life back into context, it relaxes and excites us simultaneously as we are seduced and entranced into the world from whence we emerged.

According to a BTO 2019 report, the UK population spends an estimated £200–300 million on bird feed each year, enough to feed 196 million birds![34] We crave the proximity of wildness in our lives, we yearn for some sign of connection and love and beauty, and wonder at the majesty of wild, vulnerable garden birds.

The concepts laid out within this book are my attempt to articulate some of these magical, mysterious encounters and how they can serve us in terms of our health, wellbeing, and, importantly, our sense of who and what we are: our fundamental connection to all of life beyond the labels and cultural definitions of self. This hopefully will lead us to be more caring and loving towards Nature in return, as our collective survivals are inextricably linked. Caring for Nature in this context means more than just setting aside a reserve, or feeding the birds in winter, it's an invitation to release our cultural armouring of technological separation, invulnerability, false sophistication, and abstract morality, and just surrender to the sweet memory of unity, the untamed, uncaged bird inside us.

I am not a scientist or an academic; I am an amateur (from the Latin *amare*, 'to love'). I have a deep abiding passion and love of Nature that has been with me all my life, and with that love comes sensitivity, curiosity, and a strong desire to be protective. A responsibility to fiercely defend Nature if necessary. I have sought to understand Nature from my first-hand encounters long before I discovered Goethe's 'Zarte Empirie', his 'delicate empiricism', which exhorts us to trust our bodies in this participatory dance, to feel how the body responds, and to look for evidence of the divine/intelligence within the fabric of creation, to peek behind the puppet-master's curtain. I am instinctively inquisitive about all things in life, and what happens when we consciously or otherwise tumble into that immersive experience – what is revealed to us there?

The bullfinch story complements the narrative that started with the Curlew Dance; it exemplifies Natures' ability to affect our consciousness, that even if we are not out in some vast wilderness, we are still participants in the miracle, lifted from our moribund realities and worries, and transported to another realm, a realm where we once again become like children, awestruck with the wonder of life and subsumed in the quintessence of the Universe. It is this deep, magical immersion experience that I have sought to ponder and explore in more detail throughout this book.

Forest bathing or *shinrin-yoku* is a relatively recent attempt to understand how immersion in Nature (particularly forests) can affect our physiology and psychology. There is now a burgeoning body of research and evidence for the beneficial medical impacts of being close to or observing Nature. We don't need to live in a forest to feel these benefits; just the brief encounter with the bird or a glowing cloud formation at dusk, a butterfly on the window pane, a flower, or a dawn chorus can have this transcendental effect, and these 'invitations' or affordances from Nature are always there all around us, all of the time – we just need to show up (wake up) to that unconditional love within the gesture.

Another theme worth exploring is to look at how Nature is beautiful whether we turn up or not. If I hadn't looked out the window, the bullfinch would still be as majestic as ever. Nature has its own agenda and it gets on with things regardless of whether we are there to witness it or not. Birds carry on being birds, plants carry on being plants, and rocks carry on being rocks independent of our presence, which I think is an important point to consider, as we can tend to oscillate between rampant anthropocentrism and scientific detachment. My own rather intimate adult initiation into this perspective as described in the Introduction was a complete epiphany in my deeper understanding of the relationship between Nature and *Homo sapiens*, a rite of passage delineating between my childhood, complete flow-state absorption in Nature, and the emerging adult, grappling with hormones, mystic states, and consciousness experiences.

Above all, my intention is for this to be a practical manual describing some of the ways in which we can support ourselves and others to move a little closer to this mystery, and to swap our preoccupation with consumption, preservation, and safety for a life where Nature becomes a constant companion, a wise teacher, and a path for accessing the heart, and our own innate wisdom: the Savage Self. This is the part of us that is still feral, wild, and untethered, the part that dates back to the beginning and instinctively senses the truth and is comfortable with the privilege of the unknown, and much, much more besides.

CHAPTER 3

Nature, Philosophy, and Disconnection

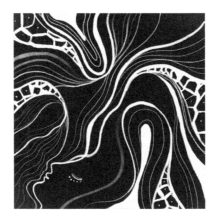

Panpsychism, monism, hylozoism, animism, and Taoism

The above terms are largely interchangeable; all describe a Universe where every part is alive and therefore has agency, where there is no separation of matter and energy/consciousness. Just as it is important to go back to the origin of everything in the known Universe from our current point of under-standing, so now we will explore the origin of our sense of separation and superiority from Nature. If we understand the genesis of this split, then we can begin to heal the tectonic divide and pull the divergent paths back to one.

Thales of Miletus (*c.* 624–545 BCE) was a pre-Socratic natural philosopher who had a massive influence on ancient Greek thought. Known as one of the seven sages of Greece, he was an astronomer, mathematician, and philos-opher, and he established the Ionian or Milesian school of philosophy, the first in ancient Greece. One of his most profound contributions to Western thought was to interrogate the origin of all things. Up until Thales' time, it was understood that the source and foundations of the natural world and all its phenomena were attributed to the myths surrounding the pantheon of gods.

By applying *logos* (logic), rather than *mythos* (story), Thales sought to distinguish natural objects and phenomena from myths, superstitions, and beliefs, and to find evidence for a common unifying energy of all matter. Thales had to separate naturalism from non-naturalism – to liberate himself from the constraints of Greek mythology, and beliefs that all life events were mediated by the presence of various gods. Thales was attempting to discover the 'substrate'. He believed that all life started with an 'originating principle' (*arche* in ancient Greek). Based on his observations of flow and dynamic properties, he proposed that all matter was derived from a single material substance: water.[35]

Outside of Vedanta, this is an early example of the philosophy of monism, the belief that all things have a common unity of origin, to which they must return, with no separation between substance and essence. Arche is an interesting word which has no direct translation, but means something like the beginning, original, or primary principle or nature/essence of a thing (the word 'archaic' is derived from it). From observing the actions and movements of magnets, Thales believed that all matter was alive, and therefore had a soul. Aristotle wrote: 'Thales thought all things are full of gods.'[36] What Thales and these early philosophers were attempting to do was to discover a common substance or essence from which all material life was derived, a preoccupation of scientists ever since.[37]

Thales and his early followers can be considered as hylozoists, *those who think all matter is alive*, and I thoroughly concur with this view. It seems evident to me that all matter and life is suffused with the originating and interpermeating essence and spirit of an intelligence that manifests in myriad forms, including us, each part revealing a facet or a microcosm of the whole.

Thales asked a question – and it is the question we need to ask whenever we venture into the wild – what is the nature and character of this energy and how it manifests as matter? How does this phenomenon uniquely demonstrate the essence of a Universal force, a form of supreme plan or calculation? (Taoists call this force Tao; see Chapter 5, Oriental Philosophy.)

Matter and energy are not separate; all matter is made of energy. $E = mc^2$: energy equals mass (matter) x the speed of light squared. At the most basic level, this equation says that energy and matter are interchangeable; they are different forms of the same thing. Under the right conditions, energy can become matter, and vice versa. We might not necessarily see it this way – how can a beam of light and a tree be different forms of the same thing? – but Nature does. When we can see all life as a manifestation of energy, we can then have deeper insight into how we are healed by spending more time with Nature. Each individual expression of that form has a corresponding different energy signature. The cells of a tree or a fungus are the genetic brothers and sisters of the bacteria and animal cells inside us.

Those early philosophers also asked: how does a plant or animal know how to be its unique self? How is a thing born with an imprint of its being already innate? How do *we* know how to be congruent with the animal self inside? If we don't know who we are, how can we know if what we are doing is aligned with our soul's purpose or journey?[38] If you don't believe in the soul, feel free to insert another term (e.g., essence, psyche, vital force, inner self). This notion of a journey to discover the soul's purpose is approaching a substantive definition of therapy in its purest form. This enquiry also leads us back to the truth of Unity, a non-dualistic Universe[39] which is an interplay of all energies at once as one indivisible expression in flow.

Thales had travelled extensively in Egypt, and his philosophical ideas had been hugely influenced by ancient Egyptian culture and cosmology. The creation myths of many early Near East civilisations including Sumerian and Babylonian regarded life as originating from water, the Cosmic Ocean. Tiamat is the Mesopotamian goddess of the sea, the symbol of the chaos of cosmic creation. In Hebrew, Tehom is considered the mythological primaeval ocean and the precursor to biblical cosmological images of the flood, which also appears in Sumerian myths. In the Bible, the book of Genesis also equates Tehom with the deep:

And the earth was without form, and void;
and darkness was upon the face of the deep.
And the Spirit of God moved upon the face of the waters.[40]

Compare this also with the *Rig Veda*, one of the original Hindu scriptures:

Darkness there was at first, by darkness hidden;

Without distinctive marks, this all was water;
That which, becoming, by the void was covered;
That One by force of heat came into being.[41]

It is evident that water was widely considered the source of all life in these ancient civilisations. Thales was partly correct, and life on Earth probably did start in a thermic vent somewhere with the right combination of heat, minerals and water. (So often we can find that myth and logic are distinct ways of describing the same phenomena; for example, the ancient Indian Vedic texts predicted the existence of the quantum field 10,000 years ago.)[42]

After a meeting with the famous Indian poet Rabindranath Tagore, Heisenberg stated:

> After these conversations (with Tagore) about Indian philosophy, some of the ideas of Quantum Physics that had seemed so crazy suddenly made much more sense.[43]

Neils Bohr said, 'I go to the Upanishad to ask questions.'[44]

Schrödinger was a lifelong student of Vedanta, and the Upanishads heavily influenced his work on quantum theory. 'There is obviously only one alternative,' he wrote, 'namely the unification of minds or consciousnesses. Their multiplicity is only apparent, in truth there is only one mind. This is the doctrine of the Upanishads.'[45] In his books *What is Life?* and *My View of the World*, he expounded on his thoughts that individual consciousness is only a manifestation of a larger unitary consciousness pervading the Universe, and 'cannot be accounted for in physical terms, for consciousness is fundamental'.[46] I fully concur with this notion, and it has also been my experience, when in an elevated state of consciousness, that ego creates separation and dualism in the mind.

Schrödinger purported a non-dualist perspective and was a fan of the Hindu idea of *tat tvam asi* from the Chandogya Upanishad verse 6.9.4 which translates as 'Thou art that' or 'That's how you are', or 'This is you', or as my good friend Geordie Dave says: 'Everything is everyone...and everything changes as we all move forward.' I really like this explanation as it summarises the two faces of the paradoxical nature of life contemplated by those early Greek philosophers

– everything remains constant, and everything is constantly changing. Every thing is connected, everyone is everything, and everything is ONE. 'The total number of minds in the Universe is one.'

> Hence this life of yours which you are living is not merely a piece of the entire existence, but is in a certain sense the whole; only this whole is not so constituted that it can be surveyed in one single glance. This, as we know, is what the Brahmins express in that sacred, mystic formula which is yet really so simple and so clear: Tat tvam asi, this is you. Or, again, in such words as 'I am in the east and in the west, I am below and above, I am this whole world'.

> Thus you can throw yourself flat on the ground, stretched out upon Mother Earth, with the certain conviction that you are one with her and she with you. You are as firmly established, as invulnerable as she, indeed a thousand times firmer and more invulnerable. As surely she will engulf you tomorrow, so surely will she bring you forth anew to new striving and suffering. And not merely 'some day': now, today, every day she is bringing you forth, not once but thousands upon thousands of times, just as every day she engulfs you a thousand times over. For eternally and always there is only now, one and the same now; the present is the only thing that has no end.[47]

So we again encounter this theme of surrender, and of being present, being totally in our embodied presence – we, here, now, One. In the forest, the sweet calling back to this state is amplified by our feelings of containment and sensory re-attunement, and subtle primitivising of self.

I think it is also worth bearing that in mind, because we humans have this knack of unconsciously calling on ancient memories (arche-types, etc.) completely unbeknownst to our conscious minds, and of course we seek to merge and return to be held by the source of all – by the Mother of all creation.

Thales' student, Anaximander (*c.* 610–546 BCE), discounted his teacher's concept that all life derived from water, due partly to his observations of fire, suggesting that the origin and building blocks of life is a substance called *apeiron*, meaning without ends, without limits or boundaries. Anaximander proposed the view that all life arose from apeiron and was destined to return to it at death. Apeiron was a divine and perpetual primordial chaos from which all things have their genesis, and also their ultimate decay, because all things originate from the indefinite to become definite and eventually return. Apeiron is also synonymous with ideas of the Universe originating in Chaos. These early pre-monotheistic attempts to give meaning to the origin and unifying force of Nature not only bear many resemblances to the Tao, but also can be traced all the way through to Einstein's theories of relativity.

The mythical primordial forces of the Universe were thought to be constructed of the four elements: Fire, Earth, Air, and Water. Apeiron also describes the concept of opposites: night and day, hot and cold, dry and moist. From these basic principles, all complexity within the world emerged. Anaximander moved science forward, away from mythic and superstitious, non-naturalistic beliefs of his predecessors. He claimed that Nature is ruled by laws, just like human societies, and anything that disturbs the balance of nature does not last long.[48]

> We can see apeiron in action when we come into the forest. One of the first things we notice is the smell of the forest: this is composed of living matter, the scent of the trees and herbs, and also the decaying vegetation, the petrichor, and the geosmin, life returning back to the source at death. This is worth an entire meditation whilst sitting still in the woods. This is reciprocity in action.

Everything was considered a subtle balance of two equal powers, which later contributed towards the creation of the Four Cardinal Virtues of Plato's *Republic*. Greek philosophy was now relating human virtues and values as arising from Consciousness, which itself arose from Nature. Compare this with excerpts from the *Tao Te Ching*:

When all the world understands beauty to be beautiful, then ugliness exists.
When all understand goodness to be good, then evil exists.
Thus existence suggests non-existence;
Easy gives rise to difficult;
Short is derived from long by comparison;
Low is distinguished from high by position;
Resonance harmonises sound;

After follows before.[49]

This reminds me of the yin-yang symbol of life containing opposites within opposites. Arche and apeiron correspond to many East Asian ideas on the origin, composition, and purpose behind life. The Taoist concept of an all-permeating, boundless, indefinable energy called Tao reflects similar attempts to understand the natural world and learn from its laws. Here is the *Tao Te Ching* again:

> Tao produces them (all things);
> Virtue feeds them;
> All of them appear in different forms;
> Each is perfected by being given power.
> Therefore none of the numerous things does not honour Tao and esteem virtue.[50]

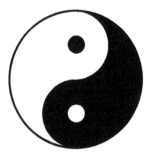

YIN-YANG.

The core teaching of the *Tao Te Ching* is an invitation to observe and learn from Nature, and that by following the wise, resourceful ways of Nature (Tao), our lives can be more aligned with healthy outcomes, and in less conflict with ourselves, each other, and with Nature. We are more *in flow*, another recurring theme. The above passage relates to this notion of balance in terms of not being attached to outcomes and seeking neither praise nor solace from others, nor ownership of anything emanating from you; don't try to depend on things, or possess things; let them go and you won't lose them (which also loosely corresponds to the Buddhist teachings of impermanence and how suffering is caused by clinging on to things).

The early Milesian philosophers were engaged in deducing the energy of life from non-supernatural forces and were commenting on the dynamism of Nature through their observations of the qualities of Earth, Water, Air, and Fire. It is this dynamic quality of Nature into which we must surrender ourselves as then we are in an alchemical process of transformation and change. Things must die, be composted down, and new things are reborn, yet everything has its own unique essence. Interestingly, those early quantum scientists such as Max Born also regarded the elementary particles as different manifestations of the same 'Primordial substance'.

The most famous disciple of Anaximander is Anaximenes (*c*. 545 BCE), who proposed that the primordial substance or arche derived from air. He called it *aer*, meaning vapour or mist. He reasoned that air in different concentrations was responsible for all life, based on his observations of cloud formations, rainbows, and phosphorescence. All life and even the Earth itself appeared from condensation and rarefaction, different densities of air. He also regarded fire as a manifestation of highly charged air, and he coined the term *pneuma* to mean breath of life. Pneuma was the infinite ever-moving divine breath that made the Universe, and aer was what humans breathed in a different density. The Bible also refers to this breath of life: 'And the LORD God formed man of the dust of the ground, and breathed into his nostrils the breath of life; and man became a living soul.'[51, 52]

Disconnection from Nature

We have now been introduced to the considerations of each of the four elements if we can accept Earth as being the prima facie divinity of the earliest pre-Hellenic tribes, and discussing the four elements in our work warrants a small chapter of its own. These early thinkers believed that the four elements would harmoniously, naturally settle into their own order when conditions were right, from which life could then advance. It is important to remind ourselves that these early Greek philosophers were animists and hylozoists (although that term wasn't created until 1678 by English clergyman and Platonic philosopher Ralph Cudworth), believing every part of life to be either alive, sentient or containing a soul, or as an expression of a larger unseen force or intelligence.

The foundations of our contemporary Western views, beliefs, and cultural values regarding Nature stem from these early attempts at understanding, and it is possible to trace how we have allowed our connection to drift apart through the later loss of spirit within science, and that separation in our minds between spirit and matter. At best we have been reduced to the false images and anthropomorphic projections of Nature that start with cuddly toys and cartoon animals that speak and never eat each other, let alone mate and defecate and fight or shed blood.

The early Greeks understood the cosmos to be a unified living organism, rather than a mechanical system. This meant for them that all its parts had an innate purpose to contribute to the harmonious functioning of the whole... The view of the cosmos as an organism also implied for the Greeks that its general properties are reflected in each of its parts. This analogy between macrocosm and microcosm, and in particular between the Earth and the human body, was articulated most eloquently by Plato in his *Timaeus* in the 4th century BCE.[53]

Plato called the universal spiritual force the Anima Mundi in his philosophical treatise *Timaeus* on the origins and workings of the Universe:

Thus, then, in accordance with the likely account, we must declare that this Cosmos has verily come into existence as a Living Creature endowed with soul and reason...a Living Creature, one and visible, containing within itself all the living creatures which are by nature akin to itself.[54]

Plato regarded the world to be endowed with a soul, in much the same way as he saw the human body having a corresponding soul which is eternal and remains alive after the person dies. This world–soul concept is borrowed from much older mythic sources but refers to a harmonious order governing the laws of life on Earth in all its forms. Order and beauty are aspects of the endless variety of life expressing itself. It is worth noting that the Latin term Anima Mundi is feminine.

Anima Mundi has its contemporary iteration in the systems-based scientific modelling of the Earth by James Lovelock and Lynn Margulis called the Gaia theory, after the ancient Greek goddess of the Earth. The Gaia model views the Earth as an intelligent self-regulating homeostatic organism, and life as the property of the planet rather than individual organisms.[55]

Plato described the Universe as being modelled by a craftsman or artisan (Demiurge), and this activity created two distinct levels of existence, the divine and the mundane. Between Anaximenes and Plato, Democritus had already stated that all matter was composed of atoms, and so we move closer to a world divided by the seen and the unseen, a world limited or restricted by the limitations of our senses, and the coincidental emergence of a new written language based not around our sensory experience of the world, but mental concepts and theories, and invisible ghost actors. By creating this notion of a two-tier system where only certain actors have access to the higher frequencies, we see the early foundations for a religion characterised by an unseen, abstract, all-powerful, and judgemental deity, dismantling the previous fusion of the practical and the sacred.

> Earlier spoken onomatopoeic languages reflect this indivisible fusion of the pragmatic and the spiritual, and our lives are then purely mediated by the daily rhythms of being. Traces of these archaic words show up in our everyday language as remnants of our pre-patriarchal-domination past.
>
> In the language of Jesus, Aramaic, the word for bread, breath, and spirit are all one; hence, 'give us this day our daily bread' from the Lord's Prayer refers to all three as one; and the intonation of the Aramaic words physically draws spirit deep into the body with the breath.
>
> To breathe is to inspire, to draw the spirit into you. Inspire is defined as:
>
>> Middle English *enspire*, from Old French *inspirer*, from Latin *inspirare* 'breathe or blow into' from *in-* 'into' + *spirare* 'breathe'. The word was originally used of a divine or supernatural being, in the sense 'impart a truth or idea to someone'.[56]

Plato's work was the first of any philosopher to be fully recorded, and this may have contributed towards his prominence. He also left some of his teachings and dialogues as slightly ambiguous pertaining to the spiritual or metaphysical aspects of Nature, and expressed an 'ambivalence with regard to nature, or to the expressive power of the natural world'.[57]

Socrates, Plato's teacher and the protagonist in his *Dialogues*, famously declares, 'You see, I am fond of learning. Now the country places and the trees won't teach me anything, and the people in the city do. We cannot learn anything from trees.'[58] This dialogue takes place whilst Phaedrus and Socrates are sitting under the shade of a plane tree, itself a reference to Plato's nickname, so there is a playful irony in these words. This moment could be said to signal the start of the separation of rational thought from the natural world.

NATURE, PHILOSOPHY, AND DISCONNECTION

Plato described the atoms of the four elements which had been key to theories of apeiron as geometric shapes based on the Platonic solids, and he argued that the higher dimensions of the Universe were only accessible through reason. Symmetry and geometry were used to describe the underlying mathematics and order of the world. His theory of Forms began to shape the modern intellect and alienation from Nature. He sought to define existence and knowledge by that which was 'eternal and unchanging',[57] in sharp contrast to his forebears who saw life manifested in all that moved and changed. He also endeavoured to define the laws of Nature by applying intellect to Nature, rather than learning from it. Contrast this with early Oriental philosophy which rarely concerned itself with symmetry, regarding it as 'a construct of the mind, rather than a property of nature, and thus of no fundamental importance'.[59]

Plato's ideas have had far-reaching consequences on the development of Western thought, and our attitudes towards Nature have been sculpted by the clay of his ambivalent dialogues and writings. Philosophers since Plato have long argued for and against a more animistic approach to our understanding of life, which is surely the goal of both physics and philosophy. It is possible to trace an unbroken line of scientific thought built upon Platonic foundations that further drives a wedge between mind and matter, spirit and body, from Aristotle to Descartes, through to Newton, and into our modern belief that science and technology can solve all of our problems.

What we must bear in mind is that this linear route of development is only one potential path, only one evolution of technology, to the exclusion of all other forms of intellectual or organic enquiry. Why must we assume that our way is the only way? Our hubris blinds us to the possibility of multiple directions for intelligence to explore outside of the limited paradigm of Platonic-Newtonian, linear, binary thinking. Other forms of technology existed that we have lost access to, but were very much a part of the development of earlier civilisations.

Plato's student Aristotle is a colossus of science and philosophy, whose works seeded the origins of all the modern sciences. Aristotle was fascinated by Nature, investigating natural phenomena at length and observing many plants and animals. In *De Anima* (Of the Soul) Aristotle wrote that through these observations he perceived that there were three different types of soul (*psyches*): plants have a vegetative or vegetal soul, animals have an animal or sensitive soul in addition to a vegetative soul, and humans, in addition to the preceding two, also have a rational soul with an intellect (*logos*) which connects us to other forms and types of life. This is yet another step towards alienation from Nature, and a false elevation of man above Nature, which will have undoubtedly influenced René Descartes in his division between mind and matter.

Whether we can find comfort in hylozoist, animist, or panpsychist perspectives of Nature, it is important to exercise our capacity to place our own consciousness outside of our minds, and see Universal consciousness located within our cells and constituents. This is like building a muscle; it takes time and careful, regular trips to the non-urban parts of our psyche, and feeling into our animate physicality and kinship with other life forms.

In the next chapter, I will introduce the long lineage of Nature mystic writers and philosophers who have kept the smouldering embers of Nature spirituality alive through hundreds of years of suppression and Judeo-Christian antipathy towards Nature, which, alongside the rapid development of land enclosures, evictions, extinctions, and the growth of trading and the industrial-capitalist machine, have turned our attentions towards money, science, and vapid consumerism.

Poetry

The other strange thing about writing a book about Nature is that a book is simply a long zigzag of words, like a squashed spring, a linear coil of symbols that stretch out towards infinity in one direction, a procession of glyphs and codes, an abstraction of the real thing as I described earlier.

It strongly suggests a two-dimensional narrative. How can that possibly elucidate or capture the true essence of Nature where everything is happening all around us, through us and all at once, where everything is linked to every other thing through this evolutionary nexus of living expression/expansion? And not only the visible worlds but the quantum worlds too, interpenetrating all life in the Cosmos, influencing life around us, outside the abstract constraints of time and reason.

Coal was forest, limestone was tiny sea creatures, glass was rock; sunlight, water, minerals all consort to create new life forms that spend millions of years adapting, evolving, and tinkering to find their ecological niche within the Earth's rich global biocommunities. Everything (including us) is related to everything else, we are eukaryotes belonging to ancient orders of life, nothing exists in isolation, and it's impossible to convey that accurately through the modes of language that we have so far developed. Some astrophysicists now believe that our material objects and everyday conditions could not have existed in isolation and are therefore inseparable from the distant regions of the Universe. The basic unity of the Cosmos manifests itself through both the macroscopic and microscopic or subatomic scales, as predicted in the Taoist texts.

For an electron to know what to do or be, it needs to know what all the other electrons in the Universe are doing. There exists a kind of super-ecology that connects our actions and thoughts with the vastness of the gas clouds and galaxies. This vast omnipresent intelligence may seem far-fetched but Panpsychism ideas are currently gaining traction with some scientists and cosmologists.

To grasp all of this complexity fully, we need to go out and immerse ourselves in the environment, look up at the stars, lower our force fields, deactivate our perceived boundaries, and rediscover our own psycho-biological niches and relax into our Original Joy. An ultimate form of this encounter is to become aware of the cells and atoms within us and how they interact with environment; this is a state that is possible to achieve with the support of certain entheogens, fevers, meditation practices, or spontaneous states of awe and grace.

So, you may be wondering why am I bothering to attempt to write a book on Nature with all the above in mind, when basically all of life is a massive entangled mess of threads, synaptic nodes and webs, and interweaving trillions of unique possibilities for random, chaotic encounters, journeys, and synchronicities – a nexus of potentialities impossible to capture. I don't know the answer, but if you need a neat, linear, carefully and methodically laid-out argument I'm afraid to disappoint you, this may not be the book for you. We are jumping around all over the place, going back on ourselves, like a fox laying a false trail, repeating certain parts, contradicting certain parts, and avoiding some black holes altogether.

If we can accept those limitations and that the book is not the territory, just a scrawled map by an inquisitive explorer, then I hope to stimulate thought, signpost towards positive Nature connection practices, and perhaps engender some feelings or responses to the words and ideas that I present (hopefully not a brick through my window, but maybe an email). Regard these words as an invitation to go deeper and more tenderly into the mystic.

My modest attempts to pass on my observations and arbitrary thoughts must be taken with the guidance that this is not a comprehensive description of all that surrounds and influences us, just a flashlight shining on a few of the parts worthy of further exploration and curiosity.

Apart from books being a linear text, the other issue is the power of words and language to distort and control the narrative. Even the medium itself can be problematic; using English has issues, translating words and losing meanings is tricky, Western-centric idioms, syntax, etymologies, cultural misappropriation, exclusion from the conversation of cultures with different language structures, and the omission of learning through other forms all present issues that the author has in mind. Basically, it's best if we just all go out in the woods and connect up in the 'field' of consciousness, the field of infinite possibility, and communicate non-verbally. I will meet you there.

However, aside from my idealistic fantasy, *if* we need to put words down, *if* we really want to edge closer to that vitality, chaos, and splendour, we can do no better than to resort to poetry. Poetry is a way of playing with the forms, the sounds, the shapes, and the smell of things.

Good poetry challenges conventions and rules, loosens things up. Poetry resonates inside the hollow trunk of the yew, and floats skyward on the hum of the bees and the song of the vixen in the night. Poetry's job is to take us beyond the established and habitual confines of the word and the mind, and drop us unprepared into the liminal space, in much the same way as *shinrin-yoku* can take us out of our habitual responses to a familiar piece of woodland or a daily walk through the fields. Poetry can lift us from the mundane and elevate our thoughts far beyond our daily consciousness, just like my bullfinch guests.

Good poetry asks us questions or poses dilemmas and unsettles our cosy perceptions. Poetry seduces us towards the in-between place, where we can be a different version of ourselves, and maybe a bit sad, rebellious, joyous, irreverent, or a feeling that defies definition. Good poetry adds nobility to our struggles and articulates those rare encounters with the wild side. I integrate poems into my *shinrin-yoku* walks, but choose poems that ask questions and leave things unanswered, or ambiguous, like the haikus, or the metaphysical poetry of David Whyte and Rainer Maria Rilke. Sometimes a poem is a great punctuation point on a walk, and can move us deeper into silence and con-templation, or be the counter-point to our wanders.

George Santayana described poetry as 'that subtle fire and inward light which seems at times to shine through the world and to touch the images in our minds with ineffable beauty'.[60]

CHAPTER 4

Phantasiai: Philosophy, Mysticism, and Reconnection

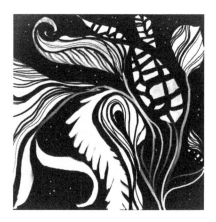

Philosophy (from the Greek *philos* 'love of', and *sophos*, 'wisdom', which possibly references Sophia the Goddess of wisdom) means love of wisdom – it's worth bearing that in mind as we move forward in our epistemological exploration, starting back with Plato and the use of language.

The new Greek alphabet revolution changed the language that Plato used to become the first language in the world not to be derived from an oral language. Oral languages by their nature tended to be onomatopoeic languages – where the sounds were mimicking the objects themselves, utterances and gestures conveying the bodily feelings of the experience, or phenomena. The new Greek language enabled Plato to expound on ideas of separation and abstraction, because the language was detached and abstract.[61]

Plato represented the Cosmos as a two-tier system where phenomena (like beauty) manifested in Nature were considered part of a transient, temporal reality that was a reflection or expression of a larger, infinite, and invisible essence beyond the range of most mortals' sensory awareness. This separation of matter and essence led inexorably towards hierarchical cultural development that left us open to persuasion and manipulation, to emulation and prostration.

Gradually, the collective 'nous' of our primal earth-based Palaeolithic and early Neolithic forebears which bound language to connection to Earth, Nature, the body – both as sound box and phenomena – was replaced by the new confident language of reason, rationality, and science. Plato was indeed suspicious of language and distanced himself from the '*Sophists*' (travelling speakers, orators, and poets), in his rejection of myths and poetry as superstitions rather than the reserves of wisdom.

The old mimetic language of embodied consciousness gave way to the new language of virtues, and beliefs in the ideas of the intelligible world; an abstract world of eternal and invisible forms not subject to corporeal temporality but existing in pure states beyond our sensorial reach, beyond sight. We sacrificed our ancient goddesses and gods on the first fires of our newfound youthful swagger and *braggadocio.*

The justification for this shift in thought and behaviour was partly to create a new class of intelligentsia invested in a language where pure reason was separate from the natural world, thus creating a kind of false objectivity which divided thinking from feeling. Greek language had neither a visual (like Chinese) nor oral semantic connection for its adherents. Our entire Western civilisation is founded on this new Greek system of literacy, and the symbols of the alphabet.

Socrates' declaration that 'the trees can't teach me anything' then epitomises this new paradigm of what B. Farrington referring to Francis Bacon calls 'intellectual pride, manifested in the presumptuous endeavour to conjure knowledge of the nature of things out of one's own head, instead of *seeking it patiently* in the Book of Nature'.[62]

This seeking patiently is absolutely key not only to the success of forest bathing integrity and depth, but also to establishing a new re-energisation of subjective empirical observation as a means of understanding life/Nature (see Goethe's *zarte Empirie*), a reversal of the mechanistic viewpoint in science and philosophy that fetishises objectivity. Plato regarded the human body as a plant rooted in heaven, with our soul or *Daemon* near the top of the body, 'and which raises us – seeing that we are not an earthly but a heavenly plant'.[63]

The introduction of this distinction has really caused so much damage, and the inversion of rootedness literally cuts us off from the ground that had up until then been our bread, breath (*Psyche*) and spirit. Contrast Plato's statement with this observation by D.H. Lawrence in his *A Propos for Lady Chatterley's Lover*:

> Man has little needs and deeper needs. We've fallen into the mistake of living from our little needs til we have lost our deeper needs in a sort of madness. Let us prepare now for the death of our little life and re-emergence in a bigger life in touch with the moving cosmos. We must get back into relation through daily ritual. We must practice again the daily ritual of dawn and noon and sunset, of kindling fire and pouring water, for the truth is, we are perishing for lack of fulfillment of our greater needs. We are cut off from the great sources of our inward nourishment and renewal. Sources that flow eternally in the universe. **Vitally the human race is dying. It is like a great uprooted tree with its roots in the air. We must plant ourselves again in the universe.**[64]

In order to now seek this re-alignment with vital life, with the moving Cosmos, how can we plant ourselves again in the Universe? I will endeavour to give some pointers towards this act of re-enchantment, towards the conversations between the soul and the whole arching firmament of the sky, the deep thrumming Earth, and the myriad miracles of Nature who offer us their company on a daily basis. Without denying the vital importance of scientific determinism and endeavour through the centuries, I will now focus on a parallel path to the lineage of reasoning, logic, and the scientific enquiries of Galileo, Francis Bacon, René Descartes, Newton and others, all the way up to the present day.

Early Nature mystic writers

Let us explore what feels like a hidden, yet unbroken lineage of Nature mystic writers, stretching back to Aristotle and forward to the present day; to writers like John O' Donahue, Nan Shepherd, Mary Oliver, David Whyte, and others who have found simple truths in the shape of the clouds and the currents of a mountain stream. Good Nature mystic writing can help to guide us along the path that others have taken, reassuring us that we are not alone; it can be transformative too, perhaps serving to boost our experiences and revelations.

> I may have missed some important players and misconstrued key turning points in our history, but the purpose is to discover universal

references and observations from our struggles, with Nature and wellbeing at the core. I want to acknowledge the primarily Western focused references in this book, and welcome the voices of indigenous wisdom from around the world. I hope that my experience will have some general similarities in its approach; what is key here is how we as a global community take back our birthright: our connection to Nature as a source of spiritual sustenance, and Nature's embrace of us as children.

The current renaissance in Nature writing is often dominated by white middle-class males, and some may lump me in that category (I am at least working class according to my daughter), but I welcome the voices of all people into this equation; we have so much to learn from each other. I would be appalled to think of forest bathing as yet another white middle-class elitist distraction. It has to be real, functional, grounded, and, if political, then about access to the countryside for all, without discrimination, and a central re-deifying of Nature as a universal principle or movement.

I therefore wish to apologise for any ignorance on my part and for what may seem a biased perspective. I welcome your voices and inputs into this arena and how we can blend our cultures to enrich our lives and understanding of our shared natural heritage. Please contact me with any kind suggestions. I can also recommend some emerging nature writers like Jini Reddy's book *Wanderland*, and *The Grassling* by Elizabeth-Jane Burnett is a poetic exploration of the countryside around Devon where I live. Both authors touch on themes that are prevalent in this book.

The earliest mystic writers are regarded from a Christian perspective, as adopted and co-opted into a view that subjugates Nature under God. However, reading between the lines, we can see that it was Nature that really moved them – they just didn't want to get thrown on a fire! Nature mysticism is an entirely different experience wherein the vast number of recorded experiences are portraying a sense of merging, of 'unselfing', becoming one with all life, dissolving into the infinite connection with all beings; Nature is sufficient alone to possess and transmit this ineffable quality of Oneness. If we can read the works of these Christianity-associated writers and replace the word God with Nature, we then have a vividly different perspective on these experiences.

One of the earliest and most remarkable writers was Hildegard of Bingen, a Benedictine abbess who was also a composer, philosopher, mystic, visionary, medical writer, and practitioner. She was a dynamic woman and an early ecologist with some profound insights into Nature. Writing in the 12th century CE, she said: 'Everything that is in the heavens, on earth, and under the earth is penetrated with connectedness, penetrated with relatedness.' Demonstrating an understanding of panpsychism, and in an extremely poignant and apposite prediction for the future, she also wrote:

> The earth should not be injured. The earth should not be destroyed. As often as the elements, the elements of the world are violated by ill treatment, so God will cleanse them through the sufferings, through the hardships of mankind.

I think that translates as us bringing down our own demise or suffering through careless actions.

Meister Eckhart, a theologian, mystic, and philosopher (*c*. 1260–1328) was accused of heresy and tried by the Papal court, but died before he received the verdict. His Wikipedia entry says he has acquired a status as a great mystic within contemporary popular Spirituality. His poem 'When I Was The Forest' is reproduced in full in Chapter 13, The Savage Self, and his writing has a deep level of humility and love for Nature. The philosopher Arthur Schopenhauer was influenced by Eckhart and compared his writings with the teachings of the Vedas and Buddhism:

> If we turn from the forms, produced by external circumstances, and go to the root of things, we shall find that Sakyamuni and Meister Eckhart teach the same thing; only that the former dared to express his ideas plainly and positively, whereas Eckhart is obliged to clothe them in the garment of the Christian myth, and to adapt his expressions thereto.[65]

I don't believe in all that Eckhart says, but he is a source of perspectives that relate to our Nature mysticism quest; he suggests that we need to discover the reality of Nature by going beyond appearances to the very essence of Nature.

The Romantic era

Further along this trail, I discovered the work of Johann Wolfgang von Goethe (1749-1832). Goethe was an early proto-phenomenologist, and his *Aphorisms on Nature* take some getting used to, but once again they share a deep heartfelt connection to Nature, beyond just passing appreciation and reflection.

Goethe was not only a writer, poet, and playwright, but as a biologist he formulated a theory of *Naturphilosophen,* contemporaneous with Darwin's *Origin of Species.* Goethe felt the 'mother earth' was alive and could generate new organisms, and his revolutionary *zarte Empirie* or 'delicate empiricism' methods of observation border on the spiritual, suggesting our own participation within creation rather than simply being detached objective observers.

> Goethe's practice of science shares with phenomenology a participatory, morally responsive, and holistic approach to the description of dynamic life-world phenomena. Delicate empiricism has its own version of the phenomenological epoché…it strives to disclose the essential or archetypal structure of the phenomenon through the endowment of human imagination.[66]

Goethe himself wrote, 'In nature we never see anything isolated, but everything in connection with something else which is before it, beside it, under it and over it',[67] echoing the panpsychist and hylozoist perspectives of Hildegard before him, and Taoist beliefs from the 4th century BCE.

Rainer Maria Rilke (1875–1926) has written much inspirational and thought-provoking poetry that bears comparison with some of Rumi's writings. Both writers have a lyrical way of invoking thought and reflection, and their prose is almost koan-like. Rilke's collection of poems translated by Joanna Macy and Anita Burrows entitled *Letters to a Young Poet* is a useful place to start. Many of Rilke's poems allude to the liminal world and are almost like verses from the *Tao Te Ching* in their use of ephemeral imagery and ambiguous spiritual language; they are so beautiful and haunting to read.

I recommend Rilke as a part of Nature connection practice. The transcendent language speaks of the solitude and existential musing of life, the seeking of solace in symbols and gestures of love, grace, and redemption. One of his stanzas, almost homoerotic in its feel, reminds me of Eckhart:

> Often when I imagine you
> your wholeness cascades into many shapes.
> You run like a herd of luminous deer
> and I am dark, I am forest.[68, 69]

We could now go in many different directions. For example, there have been calls to re-evaluate William Wordsworth's poetry as being that of a mystical writer, and certainly his ode to the River Wye, 'Lines Composed a Few Miles above Tintern Abbey', has similar imagery, evoking a sense of return, of yearning beyond conscious recourse. He invokes the motif that we suffer alone and then come back to where we belong, finding there the quality of a bigger

Nature, a grander feeling of spacious love and acceptance, here epitomised by the iconic, magical, charismatic river that I hold so close to my heart, and with which I have had many mystic moments beyond language and logic, the Wye.

> In darkness and amid the many shapes
> Of joyless daylight; when the fretful stir
> Unprofitable, and the fever of the world,
> Have hung upon the beatings of my heart –
> How oft, in spirit, have I turned to thee,
> O sylvan Wye! thou wanderer thro' the woods,
> How often has my spirit turned to thee![70]

As we begin to work with others in our forest bathing and Nature therapy practice, it is useful to build up a library of quotes, poems, and writings from many different perspectives that we can incorporate into our walk leadership repertoire. Remember to query any impulses to seek out only sugary-sweet invocations, and look to some that are more challenging or ambiguous and have a broad mix of opinions and insights. Sometimes an anti-Nature sentiment can be a powerful tool for debate and evaluation.

It is so personal, however – what speaks to one person won't work for others. I tend to default to Mary Oliver, John O'Donohue, and David Whyte, my spiritual parents of Nature poetry and psyche. Other writers that have touched me are perhaps more obscure, but when I read something that resonates with my sense of the ineffable, I feel a warm sense of companionship, connection, and understanding.

It's the febrile attempt to capture in words a moment of distinct and concentrated reality, a rare hyper-perceptual exchange in this endless vacuum of reduced aliveness, a kind of wake-up moment that brings us back into our animal senses and essential sharpness, or cosmic juxtaposition like the work of Jarod K. Anderson.

The Stoic philosopher and Roman Emperor Marcus Aurelius wrote:

> Constantly regard the universe as one living being, having one sub-
> stance and one soul; and observe how all things have reference to

one perception, the perception of this one living being; and how all things act with one movement; and how all things are the cooperating causes of all things that exist; observe too the continuous spinning of the thread and the structure of the web.[71]

This quote comes from his *Meditations*, a book of notes in Greek that he wrote only for himself between 170 and 180 CE, and illustrates this monistic and hylozoist thread alongside his determination to believe in kindness and perseverance even when life is unpredictable or going through a hard time.

Modernism into the present

I now to turn to two important writers, the naturalist Walter Murray (1900–85)[72] and the Nature mystic Richard Jefferies (1848–87). Jefferies, the son of a farmer from Swindon, wrote novels and essays about his experiences and adventures, and his rich, detailed observations of Nature are a joy to read. There were periods when he worked as a newspaper reporter, and the majority of his later work references his earlier youth; it speaks to the soul with a sublime transcendent quality:

I cannot leave it; I must stay under the old tree in the midst of the long grass, the luxury of the leaves, and the song in the very air. I seem as if I could feel all the glowing life the sunshine gives and the south wind calls to being. The endless grass, the endless leaves, the immense strength of the oak expanding, the unalloyed joy of finch and blackbird; from all of them I receive a little. Each gives me something of the pure joy they gather for themselves. In the blackbird's melody one note is mine; in the dance of the leaf shadows the formed maze is for me, though the motion is theirs; the flowers with a thousand faces have collected the kisses of the morning. Feeling with them, I receive some, at least, of their fulness of life... These are the only hours that are not wasted – these hours that absorb the soul and fill it with beauty. This is real life, and all else is illusion, or mere endurance.[73]

Here we touch on the true purpose of Nature mysticism: to find the succour and embrace we crave to give us a greater sense of truth beyond the stories that the bruised or damaged ego tells us. We all experience death, loss, grief, sadness, rage, and depression, and yet Nature comes to us unconditionally

and salves our deepest wounds through the 'varieties of religious experience',[74] through the spiritual sublimation of our human desires and invisible
sufferings into a cosmic context that both alleviates and recalibrates our
pains, fears, and anxieties.

As Walter Murray describes, who could fail to be moved by the sight and
sound of geese migrating overhead?

> Each night in their multitudes they fly northward. Who so disinterested in
> birds but cannot feel a thrill when on some moonless April night the dark sky
> is filled with shrill cries as unseen, but clearly heard, the winged companies
> pass overhead.[75]

This in turn reminds me of Mary Oliver's soaring poem 'Wild Geese'[76] which
also picks up on this theme of finding solace and redemption in the wild living
world. I would wholeheartedly encourage the reader to read 'Wild Geese' out
loud to yourselves (maybe not in a café) right now and just feel the immense
freedom that it invites in. This poem reaches out to all of us equivocally
beckoning our wild unfettered souls to return home.

Wild Geese

You do not have to be good.
You do not have to walk on your knees
For a hundred miles through the desert, repenting.
You only have to let the soft animal of your body love what it loves.
Tell me about despair, yours, and I will tell you
mine.
Meanwhile the world goes on.
Meanwhile the sun and the clear pebbles of the
rain
are moving across the landscapes,
over the prairies and the deep trees,
the mountains and the rivers.
Meanwhile the wild geese, high in the clean blue
air,
are heading home again.
Whoever you are, no matter how lonely,
the world offers itself to your imagination,
calls to you like the wild geese, harsh and
exciting –
over and over announcing your place
in the family of things.

This 'announcing your place in the family of things' is the clarion call to come back, the call of the wild beckoning us to return from our childish fantasies of false wealth and false self; come back and join us, the chorus sings in unison, leave your folly, your seductive trance of comfort, and find the undiscovered kingdom of Nature.[77] Through these wild sounds, the voice of Nature communicates most effectively with us; these sounds are imprinted on our souls, and when the animals within us hear them, it stirs some vague memory of kinship. Murray is aware of this siren-like music and the kinship it heralds:

> ...every one of us, at almost any time, in almost any place, can with a little trying, a little quiet contemplation, find kinship with all creation... But just as some of us have no ear for great music, or fancy we have not, and must discipline ourselves to real listening before joy comes, so most of us are blunted to that fuller understanding of nature; and perhaps only by such simple experience as that of watching birds...shall we discover a kingdom, and learn the first word of its language.[78]

These recurring themes of beauty, music, language, birds, heeding the wild call, and Nature's yearning for our company can be accommodated within forest bathing and Nature therapy sessions by exploring the senses, remaining open to spontaneity, and by setting the intention to recommence this sacred dialogue, redirecting our thirsty spirits back to the beauty of life, the true effervescent beauty of being, the song of creation that (with advanced technologies) we can hear in the distant murmurs of the expanding galaxies and the electro-organic signalling of the mycelial web.

Jefferies witnessed and rejoiced in these phenomena 140 years ago:

> With all the intensity of feeling which exalted me, all the intense communion I held with the earth, the sun and sky, the stars hidden by the light, with the ocean – in no manner can the thrilling depth of these feelings be written – with these I prayed, as if they were the keys of an instrument, of an organ, with which I swelled forth the note of my soul, redoubling my own voice by their power...the inexpressible beauty of all filled me with a rapture, and ecstasy.[79]

I believe that now there is not just an opportunity to return, but that it is incumbent upon us to direct all our efforts towards salvaging the Earth from our pollution by being sensitive and mindful of our every gesture towards Nature – our home and our sanctuary. Our highest priority is to become caring and joyful with Nature before our thuggery and philosophical, academic, political, and capitalist greenwashing destroys us all.

Coincidentally, we stand at the dawn of a psychedelic renaissance, as we research how these sacred substances can be synthesised for the sole purpose of relieving the suffering of mental health disorders. Whilst this is a noble cause, this does not address the cause of the problems or acknowledge the spirits of the plants which accompany the powerful visions. Nature mysticism and psychedelic experiences share much in common in terms of their ineffability and other key factors as noted by William James.[80]

I fully believe that it is possible to achieve these visionary and ecstatic moments within Nature without recourse to drugs and entheogens, by simply retuning our senses and opening our hearts within a context of safety and holding. Let's not miss this imperative opportunity for Earth and soul sanctification. We are all Nature mystics now, stepping out into the sun and noticing.

> The Nature Mystic goes deeper down to the heart of things, and holds that to lose touch with Nature is to lose touch with reality as manifested in Nature...it is not mere lack of education of the senses... but the stunting of the soul-life that ensues on divorce from Nature, and from the great store of primal and fundamental ideas which are immanent within.[81]

Nature mysticism experiences, although usually solitary, need to be held collectively and become an important aspect of our re-enchantment work with a circular, cyclical, feminine growth/zero-waste lifestyle. Coming back to Nature heals our wounds at every level, not just physically – research has only touched on a small part of this potential. But let us also heal the rift between us and Nature by reciprocating with our prayers and songs, rather than perpetuating the appalling habit of commodifying Nature and heedlessly exploiting it to solve problems that we caused in the first place, like a spoiled child clawing at its mother's apron, demanding a cuddle when our conscience kicks in.

Thuggery

What's going on?

We are in trouble, we are in big, big trouble, both personally and globally. It is dawning on us that we may have passed the point of no return in terms of runaway climate change (we may have already failed to achieve the 1.5° limit) and the compromise of the Ecosphere.

This book didn't set out to be a polemic on the state of things, as I'm sure you are just as aware as we all are by now of the impending climate catastrophe and sixth major extinction event looming on the horizon that we are creating. Yet it feels remiss of me to simply focus on all the nice, attractive aspects of forest bathing without presenting the context and backdrop of the urgency of the environmental crisis we are currently facing as both practical, existential, and moral dilemma.

Sometimes the enormity of the situation may make us want to turn away and ignore the complex issues we face, as we realise radical solutions will demand a change of lifestyle or a significant decrease in consumption of non-renewable resources, and possibly a need for a significant rethink, a self re-evaluation, confronting the false foundations of growth, capitalism, and Cartesian duality, without falling down the deep spiral of eco-anxiety and apocalyptic doom. (See 'Suffering' and watch Greta Thunberg's full speech to the WEF.[82])

When I recently discussed with some of my students the challenges of writing a book on deep Nature, where language is relative and text is linear compared to how Nature is all chaos, flow, miracles, and fireworks, and layer upon layer of intricate multidimensional relational complexity, they said, 'Ah, it was all fractals.' Hmm...fractals don't exactly lend themselves very easily to verbal or written description; they are amazing visually, and they do very clearly mimic some Universal law that everything exists within some sort of repeating pattern at both macro (cosmic) and micro levels of life.

In that respect, the complexity of patterns and the mix of order and chaos within fractal images serves to highlight that some of the logistical challenges and limitations in a book about Nature, which attempts to accurately convey the true essence of Nature within the structure and semantics of language, is always going to leave out aspects and focus on others, in this case the notion that forest bathing can support wellbeing, but let us take it forward with equal concern and value for the relationship and the respect Nature deserves.

This book is in many ways a cri de coeur, a summoning of the ancient sprits of the land and water, and a search for the path back home. Nature is extraordinarily well conceived, constructed, and maintained, a system of such diversity and variability, and yet it all works together, from electrons to galaxies, everything balances out everything else in a dynamic interplay of mind-blowing proportions.

Life expresses itself spontaneously, and we seek meaning and patterns from that expression through the mediums and symbols of both Mathematics and Art equally.

The big problem (and you're not going to like this) is that we are basically thugs. As a species we are thugs (brutes), we are primate thugs no less, and we have taken our thuggery as far as we can possibly go, almost entirely unrestrained, everywhere on Earth. Every continent has become contaminated and colonialised by us in our pursuit of wealth, power, growth.

This is our irrepressible need to explore and exploit, and inadvertently destroy all that we encounter: we destroy forests, we destroy mountains, we destroy plants and animals, we destroy rivers and seas, we destroy the air and the ground, we destroy ecosystems, we destroy anyone within the same species that doesn't look or think like us, or who gets in the way, and then finally we destroy ourselves – how's that![83]

This thuggery and these destructive tendencies emanate from many expressions of our evolutionary development, and the argument continues about whether we have always been aggressive, or whether our current 'machismo' originated from our transition to agricultural and hierarchical societies where defence of the crops and hoarding became the norm.

Is it woolly sentimentalism and rosy retrospection? Each year we are going faster in order to stand still; we are pushing more, driving more, straining more, ignoring more, and expecting more. Articles abound online about the significant deterioration in basic manners and politeness, loss of civility replaced by boundaries. And now AI has arrived in full force as an existential threat to humanity.

Jaron Lanier asserts that the dominant ideology of the digital world has failed humanity. He writes about a spiritual failure – that these ideologies and technologies have encouraged narrow philosophies that deny (or I think suppress) the mystery of the existence of experience. This has led to our faith being directed away from people and towards gadgets. He further describes a second failure in how these emerging technologies tend to reinforce indifferent or poor (de-humanising) treatment of humans.[84]

The machines we have created are treating us with the same level of colonial contempt as we ideologically treat other beings whom we consider beneath us. Our need for dominance has been encoded within our minds, the minds which program the very machines that may be our servants or our masters.

We have more and more legislation to tell us how to behave towards others in our workplace, social environments, and at home too, but we have largely forgotten how to be gentle people. This insidious masculinising process has been escalating for quite a while, and it affects men and women both in equal but different ways. Of course, many will argue that we have descended from apes, and they tend to demonstrate the same aggressive, acquisitive, and territorial tendencies which gives us no hope; however, they also demonstrate the capacity to care and nurture and show affection. We have the innate capacity to show empathy towards others, and our current crisis is demanding that we find ways to work together as a global community, because we understand that the other way of reacting when resources become scarce is to become more hostile.

Where we need those qualities of being 'masculine' is when we are hunting down a large and potentially ferocious, dangerous beast, or when we are defending our tribe from attack. The qualities we need for those two scenarios are to be brave, strong, override our fears, de-sensitise ourselves so we are immune to pain for a while, be adrenalised, and so that we can potentially kill another being. That's the genetic blueprint for the development of aggressive masculinity, something to switch on in those extreme or acute moments. The rest of the time, native masculinity can be effectively dialled down, and we are calm, tranquil, relaxed but alert.

Unfortunately, that archetypal masculine energy has become misappropriated, the 'feminine' has become suppressed or disavowed, and everything is now out of kilter. I know I am simplifying a very complex subject, but what I see around me is a predominantly masculine society, trying to find hard masculine solutions for the distorted masculine damage to the Earth (feminine). Patriarchy is oppressive to all of us; it acts to elevate male principles and needs above the needs of women/Earth, and to subjugate the 'anarchic' and primal forces within the feminine, with a consequent loss of receptivity and care.

In our eventual transition from hunter-gatherers to agrarians, from palaeolithic to neolithic, what agriculture initiated and then industrialisation ratcheted up was to create a permanent chronic state of mobilisation, perceived threat response, and meta-anxiety. Those very same qualities of de-sensitisation that enabled us to survive and live as hunters have now become our default global M.O.[85]

In the process of colonising new lands, we also switched from an Earth-bound personal belief system based around local or tribal variations of the Goddess and other practical deities, to an out-of-reach monotheistic male religious system that further alienated us from our sense of connection and being a part of everything – belonging in Nature, rather than dominating it.

That does not mean that we should swing back over to a completely feminine society – that too would generate its own problems – but if we can just stop and observe Nature as an effective self-regulating system without political agendas, we might learn how to structure our society, just as the ancient Taoists recommended. In that respect, we would place the feminine at the heart of our decision-making processes, qualities of receptivity, inner strength, intuitive respect for life. Putting life first, prioritising Nature first in our planning. Could this ever be possible? Will this be forced upon us eventually? Is it already happening in a subtle way? This is one of the underlying themes of this book and how it informs our nature therapy practices.

Broader than that, can you just for a moment imagine a world where the principles and values associated with deep feminism drove every religion, political decision, and social structure globally. A world where women felt safe, free, and equal, a world where men could relax into their more 'sensitive' sides, where the qualities of masculinity and femininity were in balance and equally valued, the yin-yang energies, each serving and honouring the other, instead of the 'unnatural' aggressively polarising and debilitating tension we have now. Maybe this is naivety on a global scale, but the current ideology has failed totally.

The *Tao Te Ching* is the main text of Taoist philosophy and it has equally been a strong influence on the development of Shinto (the main religion of Japan) alongside Buddhism too. These two national religions have in turn had an influence on the development of *shinrin-yoku* within Japan; although this is never explicitly stated, it's implicit within the ethos of the walks, and the fact that most Shinto shrines have an enclosing area of forest surrounding them for the spirits or *kami* to live in, and these areas are often associated with *shinrin-yoku* walks.

The original *Tao Te Ching* has been dated to around the 4th century BCE in China and is attributed to Lao Tzu which means 'wise one'. The book was written as advice for leaders who were at that time almost uniquely male. That advice was clear and simple: if you want to rule well, learn to be more humble, and importantly learn from Nature – particularly learn how to honour and respect the feminine. Advice our leaders of today have lost touch with, yet it still resonates as universal sound instruction.

The Tao is the life force that permeates everything in the Universe, and it is described as being a feminine force, a force for leaders to serve in order to rule well. In one chapter, Lao Tzu suggests that good leaders should place themselves beneath the rivers[86] (so under the feminine), suggesting that in order to be respected, one has to not only learn humility but learn to be of deep service to support the flow of the Tao.

The transpersonal psychologist Rosemarie Anderson has translated the *Tao Te Ching*, restoring the original descriptions of the Tao as feminine, as the 'dark womb of creation'.[87] She talks about the Oriental concept of *wu wei*, 'doing without doing', 'effortless action', and 'a path to peace and wellbeing for the self, others and the Earth'.

Wu wei is an example of how feminist perspectives have been incorporated into a Nature-based philosophy that may seem completely alien to Western minds. *Wu wei* is not about striving to achieve; it is about being in flow with the Tao, non-resistant, responsive, spontaneous, and, above all, yielding. Compare those qualities with how most of us live our lives now. It is also not about being lazy or indifferent; quite the reverse, it is about being tuned in to each moment so that our responses are in alignment with the Tao, and therefore are in harmony with life.

Wu wei is also about the dissolution of the ego, and ego is yet another major characteristic of our celebrity-dominated culture of entitlement and status. It is as if we live in a closed society with values that arise from a very childish or immature perception of the world, that perpetuate this hubristic notion that Nature is just a set of free resources for us to plunder in the name of progress, technology, and vanity.

The father of biophilia, Edward Wilson, wrote that 'the real problem of humanity is the following: we have Paleolithic emotions, medieval institutions and godlike technology'.[88] In Part Three of *The Patterning Instinct*,[89] Jeremy Lent discusses the divide between East and West with the title: The Patterns Diverge – Western Pattern: Split Cosmos, Split Human; Eastern Pattern: Harmonic Web of Life.

The carefully observed and slowly contemplated philosophies from the East may seem restrictive or over-disciplined, but I have found that they contain great wisdom and balance, and align beautifully with my observations of natural phenomena and patterns of energy within Nature. We all need some boundaries, and a child without boundaries becomes spoilt and lost, so I think of these wise, ancient texts as a form of boundary setting or parenting, based not on a specific agenda but on the universal principles governing all existence.

This also informs our therapeutic work with clients in Nature, discovering parallel processes within Nature that represent innovative ways to express the dynamic flow of the Tao. These organic processes and forms are both literal and symbolic, and shed light on our own internal ecologies and psycho-neural processes, and contribute to therapeutic insights and change.

With regard to our integration of the deeper principles of *shinrin-yoku* into our own practice, it is worth considering these essential qualities both of Taoism and of *wu wei*. (We will discuss Taoism and Shintoism in Chapter 5.) Exploring some of the values and insights of Taoism can be useful for informing our own walk practice and how we approach leading walks and the types of questions that can arise.

Taoists regard logical reasoning, conventional knowledge, and the intellect to be untrustworthy and a manifestation of the abstract and 'artificial world of man, together with social etiquette and moral standards'.[90] Early Taoists were not interested in the world of convention but instead preferred to observe and learn from the ways of Nature in order to discern the 'characteristics of the Tao'. Their close observations in combination with their intuitive mysticism and simple existence led them to remarkable discoveries which are only now being verified by modern science.

If we are to survive, aligning ourselves with these ancient Cosmos- and Earth-observing philosophies can guide a shift in global culture towards quality over quantity, and a maturity of the collective psyche which places value on vulnerability, diversity, and beauty. At this point, we may need sound philosophy over abstract religion. Maturity and tolerance over growth and expansion, responsibility over profit and destruction. Aliveness to Nature's beauty dissolves the synthetic boundary between ourselves and the destiny of our planet.

CHAPTER 5

Oriental Philosophy

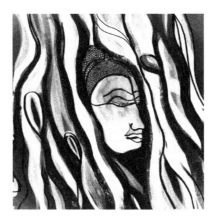

Shinto

There are two main 'religions'[91] in Japan today, Shinto and Buddhism.[92] They have existed side by side for at least 1500 years and have flourished in different ways within Japanese culture and sociopolitical interests. Shinto predates Buddhism and is regarded as the native or indigenous religion of Japan, originating from the animistic-shamanistic beliefs of the hunter-gatherer societies of the Jōmon period[93] ca. 14,000–300 BCE.

Shinto started not as a religion but as a collection of native beliefs and mythologies. The portrayal of Shinto as the ancient native 'ethnic' religion of Japan is problematical, and these early origins have been romanticised and distorted to promote patriotic sentiments towards Japanese identity and ethnicity. Shinto has been regarded as:

> The indigenous faith of the Japanese. It is a way of life and a way of thinking that has been an integral part of Japanese culture since ancient times. Shinto places great value on purity and honesty, yet as a faith, Shinto has no dogma,

doctrine, or founder. Its origins can be seen in the relationship between the ancient Japanese and the power they found in the natural world.[94]

Modern-day Shinto is a secularised version that has been associated with the political movement in Japan since 1947. Some agencies have started recently to rebrand Shinto as an environmental religion or movement.[94]

The word Shinto (*Shintō*, or *Kami no-michi*) means 'the Way of the Gods' and was originally represented as *Jindo* or *Shindo* from the Chinese *Shendao*, combining two syllables: *shen/shin* or *kami* meaning spirits and *dao* or *michi* meaning the way – the literal or metaphysical path. *Kami* are regarded as spirits, essences, gods, deities, sources of phenomena, and even sudden epiphanies may be regarded as the work of *kami*. *Kami* are in every alive component of the Universe and the sacred essence of all life.

Kami manifest themselves through the multiple forms of Nature such as rocks, mountains, trees, rivers, lakes, and animals, and even people can be said to possess *kami*. *Kami* and people are not separate; they are one, existing within the same continuum, the same world, and subject to the same laws that govern nature. *Kami* are in the Sun, the Moon, and weather, like wind and thunder. *Kami* are everywhere and share the divine complexity of all things, and Shinto shrines are established to offer prayers to various *kami* in order to achieve harmony with life. There are approximately 100,000 to 120,000 shrines left in Japan, and these shrines are generally surrounded by trees or forest.

These forest areas are called *chinju no mori* and are regarded as sacred places where the *kami* spirits like to dwell. *Chinju no mori* are central to Shinto core beliefs and values as they have represented these places of worship since ancient times. *Chinju* relates to the local deity, spirits, or *kami* and means to protect, and *mori* means forest but has come to differentiate old growth primal forest from cultivated or planted forest (*hayashi*). *Mori* refers to things in their natural state, to 'deep forest'. It carries profound symbolic capital, 'associated with notions of a spirited, non-human "other world", ancestral traditions and memories...[which] has a certain numinous, transcendent quality'.[95]

Shinto scholars point out that the etymological roots of *mori* signify both forest and sacred grove, indicating that originally it was the forest that was worshipped – the forest *was* the shrine long before specific Shinto shrines were erected. Sacred groves, such as those worshipped in Celtic and North American First Nation traditions, represent the origin of shrine worship, although the practice may be older still, originating in early African tribal rituals. The sacred forest is central not only to the origin of Shinto as an animistic belief system, but also to Japanese society as a whole[96]: the first communities constelled around these shrine-groves, and the language reflected how central the forest was to their values and culture (e.g., *shakai*, the Japanese word for society, means 'meeting in the forest'.[96])

Early Shinto pilgrims would travel large distances to observe rituals for specific purposes linked to *kami* of particular shrines: for good health, fertility, crops, etc., and some were ancestral shrines linked to particular families. These ancient pilgrimage routes have all but disappeared in modern Japan, but a few still remain, such as the Kumano Kodo in Honshu province, with the odd teahouse for the weary traveller.

Originally, these long cross-country walks may have taken days or weeks, with pilgrims often exposed to extremes of weather, and so feudal lords planted hinoki and sugi trees along the routes for shelter and protection (incidentally, the two main trees subject to the *shinrin-yoku* research in Japan). All day long, pilgrims would be breathing in the wonderful phytoncides, their pilgrimage therefore being both physically healing and a sacred journey. Hinoki and sugi trees were also most commonly used for the construction of Shinto and Buddhist temples, so again all those wonderful oils would be breathed in during temple rituals.

It is reasonable to consider that Shinto had a strong influence on the development and inspiration for *shinrin-yoku* walks, which are mini pilgrimages, not to ancient shrines *per se*, but to find the self, to restore the natural balance in each person through that immersion in the *chinju no mori*. It makes sense that this would bring us back full circle to the sacred groves of the past. The experiment of intense urban living creates casualties who must withdraw to the healing power of the deep woods.

Taoism

Taoism is not a clearly identifiable religion but is defined as a syncretic religion or philosophy, which has evolved by amalgamating shamanistic beliefs, philosophies, animistic folk practices and doctrines. At its core is the Sage, a wise woman or man quietly and patiently observing the workings of Nature and how they resonate with their own lives and with social constructs.

Lao Tzu is credited with being its founding father and Highest Venerable Master, but so much about his life is shrouded in legend that it is hard to sort the truth from the myths. Some historians have suggested that he lived somewhere between the 4th and 6th centuries BCE. His most famous book is the *Tao Te Ching*. Lao Tzu was a contemporary of Confucius, and both Taoism and Confucianism entered Japan from mainland China and Korea, where they were assimilated and integrated into the indigenous belief systems alongside Shinto. The first recordings of Taoism in Japan are in the *Nihon Shoki* around the 7th century CE.

The region of Southern China that Lao Tzu grew up in was a stronghold of shamanistic beliefs, which worshipped the Earth, Heavens, and places in Nature alongside animals like the bear, deer, birds, and fish. Lao Tzu, like Confucius, had become disillusioned with the political intrigues and ruthlessness of the feudal lords. Legend tells us that he came to some kind of enlightenment, travelled to the western frontier, and disappeared (or became immortal).[97] As he was attempting to leave the city gates, he was recognised by the Gatekeeper Wen Shih, who said that he wasn't allowed to leave until he had put all his wisdom down on paper. And so Lao Tzu created the *Tao Te Ching*. Scholars now think that it was the work of more than one person, but nevertheless it is a fundamental embodiment and treatise of all Taoist thought.

The *Tao Te Ching* offers advice to rulers and statesmen on how to conduct themselves to rule well and have happy subjects by observing the ways of Nature. As the majority of rulers at the time were constantly warring, and were mostly men, the advice suggests adopting a more receptive and feminine attitude towards life. Learning from Nature and following the energy of the Tao was regarded as beneficial for individuals and for leaders. Tao is seen as a ubiquitous force or energy that is present in all of life. Tao represents the harmony of existence within the natural order, so by aligning ourselves with the Tao, we can come into harmony with life.

The first chapter of the *Tao Te Ching* describes the all-embracing true Tao as a nameless, inexhaustible source of flow and life force. The Tao is not a deity but is present in all the myriad forms of Nature like rivers, forests, mountains, sky, and the Earth. It is similar to Shinto's concept of the *kami* or spirits which inhabit all things. The *Tao Te Ching* regards this force as benevolent: 'The Celestial Way is to benefit others and not to cause harm' (Chapter 81); and since the 'Celestial Way follows the Way of the Tao' (Chapter 25), we can assume that in the *Tao Te Ching*, the Tao is a benevolent force.[97]

I have always believed in this benevolent force, and Nature's active benignity. As a young man, it felt important to just learn from Nature and not be influenced by others' thoughts or views of Nature, so I avoided all books until I came across the *Tao Te Ching* and the *I Ching*, and I realised just how much of this made sense and offered a cohesive structure to my understanding of Nature and all its peculiarities.

There are many versions and translations of the *Tao Te Ching*, but when I read most of them, I sense that the translators have attempted to take the ambiguity and slightly riddle-like form out of the text and put too much Western explanation into it. My little falling-apart volume is a translation by Ch'u Ta-kao, published by Unwin in 1972; it leaves the wording so koan-like and poetic that it takes time to consider what each chapter means and how it opens us up to the mystery of the Universe and the workings of Nature. The main emphasis for me is the indication that leaders who follow the Tao (Sages) are humble and fully embrace the feminine energy that is inherent within the harmonious movements of Nature.

The Taoist classic, *Baopuzi* ('The Master Who Embraces Simplicity'), from the 4th century CE, makes a distinction between two kinds of people concerning their relationship with Nature: one is 'those who enslave the myriad things', and the other is 'those who emulate Nature'. Those who have only a superficial understanding of the relationship between people and Nature are the ones who 'enslave the myriad things'; they subjugate Nature completely to themselves. Contrariwise, people who have a profound insight into the mystery of the relationship between humans and Nature are friends of Nature; they derive their understanding of longevity from Nature by meditative observation and gazing.[98]

Whilst Shinto evolved from earlier pagan animistic beliefs and became assimilated into the beliefs of the indigenous tribes of Japan, and was later influenced and co-existed with incoming religious ideas like Confucianism and Buddhism, Taoism arose as a separate movement that venerated the old ways, as a reaction to the corruption within Chinese government and society around the 4th century BCE. Shinto and Taoism are very closely aligned in their respective ways of revering the capricious forces of Nature.

When I discovered the *Tao Te Ching* and started to delve into its peculiar language, what struck me so strongly was that it reflected all that I had witnessed in Nature since childhood, and described a body of thought that recognised the power and wisdom of the natural world and its phenomena in a way that I had experienced but felt largely alone with.

Taoism is for me one of the foundation stones of this work, and if one can grasp the tenets of the Tao, then leading *shinrin-yoku* walks takes on another level of meaning. In Taoism, the central concept is relationship; we cannot approach Nature as a thing to be mastered, but as a partner in a relationship. The goal is to become a natural part of the original order – the way to discover that original order is to turn to Nature.

Early Taoist philosophers left the cities to learn from Nature and primitive people living in remote mountain villages. They hoped to eventually bring human civilisation into the natural order. In Taoism, Nature is taken to be infinitely wise, infinitely complex, and infinitely irrational. One must take a yielding stance and abandon all intellectual preconceptions. The goal is *wu wei*, doing nothing contrary to Nature. Nature does not need to be perfected or improved. It is we who need to change, we need to come into accord.

Taoists rejected all dichotomies, even the most fundamental one of being versus non-being, for both come from the same source, 'at the deep and the profound'. The goal of Taoism is to attain that which precedes duality. The only way to discover this original source is to observe Nature. During peak experiences in Nature, the deep meets the deep. The Tao is a divine chaos, not a random accident. It is fertile, undifferentiated, and teeming with unrealised creation. It is the mother of everything in Nature; it is a great darkness that operates spontaneously to give birth and life to all things.

Taoists seek not to be saved or to win, but rather to return to the original source of the Ten Thousand Things. They see creation not as a single event, but an ongoing process that has no beginning and no end. Its divine play is taking place right here and right now. The wise person becomes like an animal or a child, participating joyfully in the profoundly irrational order. He or she learns to trust the chaos.

The Taoists have always avoided anthropocentrism. Unlike other religions, they have never lost their animal gods. Ancient Chinese shamans put on animal masks to communicate with these animal gods; their spirit-animals were links between the worlds of people, ancestors, and gods. There was a tradition of animal frolics during which one became a particular animal, such as a crane or a bear. These rituals are still meaningful.

Taoists speak of a direct knowing that resonates in the belly when one has direct contact with Nature. It is not with the head but with the belly that one can participate in the sacred madness of the ancestral gods. It is only with the belly that one can appreciate the eternal flux and the underlying unity of the 'Ten Thousand Things'.

The basic assumptions of Taoism[99]

- The source of Nature is spirit.
- Nature is not a random accident. It has meaning, significance, and purpose.
- Certain aspects of Nature are invisible.

- Nature is a part of a greater whole, which is beyond time and space.

- Nature's beauty has intrinsic value.

- That which preserves the beauty and harmony of Nature is good. That which destroys it is bad.

- All animals, plants, and landscapes are sacred.

- All creatures have an equal right to self-fulfilment.

- The inner world is a part of Nature.

- We should celebrate the Creation with song, dance, art, poetry, and stories.

- Science is an indispensable tool for gaining knowledge about Nature. Scientism (the belief that science is the only source of wisdom) is, however, a dangerous and misguided philosophy.

Embracing the Way, you become embraced;
Breathing gently, you become newborn;
Clearing your mind, you become clear;
Nurturing your children, you become impartial;
Opening your heart, you become accepted;
Accepting the world, you embrace the Way.
Bearing and nurturing,
Creating but not owning,
Giving without demanding,
This is harmony.[100]

Taoism is a philosophy of Flow. It is of great interest to us as forest bathing leaders as it points towards this East Asian perception of the Nature around us as not only alive and brimming with Tao energy but also offering us these deeper insights into the nature of Being into our own personal ontology and collective consciousness. It also flows wonderfully into Arne Næss's work and the Deep Ecology movement.[101] Why can't our current political leaders entertain these ideas and listen to the Sages who still exist in many societies? Hubris, I guess.

Why?

Why, why why? That's the question that I've always asked since I was an inquisitive, precocious child. My therapist would often say to me, 'Stefan, don't ask why; why is not the right question, why will just get you into trouble,' meaning that I will only tie myself in more knots by never getting a satisfactory answer, or any answer or explanation for behaviour. As a therapist myself I never directly ask why, but approach understanding and reasons behind behaviours by asking, 'I wonder why that is happening?' followed by 'I wonder when it may have first happened?', either expressed verbally or held internally.

'Why?' asks external, straightforward questions – 'Why does the Earth appear flat?' – and internal or rhetorical ones – 'Why do people do that to each other/the environment/themselves?' I asked a lot of the latter sort of questions in an attempt to understand the kinds of behaviour which have no direct basis in logic but certainly a basis in the primitive development and evolution of the early hominid. Aggression, superstition, territorial defence, and acquisitiveness I can see would all play a part in our early tribal communities and therefore be part of our genes for survival (although anthropologically there are many fine examples of first contacts with tribes without hostility and fear). I have referenced some excellent studies by philosopher Mary Midgeley to underscore these points which in some ways might seem contradictory. The idea of the noble savage is a myth born from colonialist superiority attitudes.

Asking why was the original question which challenged our ignorance of the animated cosmos that we inhabited; curiosity, and balancing fear with curiosity, is what caused our brains to grow and develop ever more complex processing abilities.

Why discovers truths below the surface and it never stops. I like why because I will never cease in my exploration and enquiry into Nature; it's endless, and that's why it has been so hard to write this book – where do you draw the line, because each of these topics goes off into infinity in every direction. What to include, what to omit? Nature asks questions of us and demands no answers.

Existential or ontological questions like 'Why are we here?', 'What is the very nature of being?', and 'How do I know that I exist?' are perennial desires for elusive answers that never come. Sometimes our perpetual sense of curiosity causes harm to the planet and perhaps we need some things to be left mysterious and unfathomable – ineffable. This quote from the wonderful *Walden* by Thoreau summarises this point well:

> We need the tonic of wildness... At the same time that we are earnest to explore and learn all things, we require that all things be mysterious and unexplorable, that land and sea be indefinitely wild, unsurveyed and unfathomed by us because unfathomable. We can never have enough of nature.[102]

Asking why can be both penetrative and introspective, speculative or focused, pertinent. Let's keep asking why, whilst also embracing the mystery of not knowing, of the unknown; let us in Gary Snyder's words 'remain unprepared'[103] and then there will be room for an answer. I also invite you to remain curious at all times in Nature, to never assume, but seek to discover first hand and maybe later learn more. What was that strange jelly substance coming out of the ground? Why is that plant covered in caterpillars? Why am I feeling so off-balance? Is there a link between x and y? Why seeks reasons, sometimes where none exist; why is both our drive for success as a species and also our downfall in missing opportunities for acceptance and peace.

I will conclude with a cheeky quote from physicist Richard Feynman: 'Study hard what interests you the most in the most undisciplined, irreverent and original manner possible.'[104]

CHAPTER 6

Fundamentals of *Shinrin-Yoku*

To evolve we need to come back into the heart, to come back into place of connection to the heart; in order for our shinrin-yoku work to evolve we need to include the heart in all that we do alongside the mind. I want to emphasise that this is not a sentimental approach, Nature is never sentimental, Nature is efficient, Nature is fierce, Nature is raucous, Nature is ebullient, Nature is rhapsodic, Nature is spectacular, Nature is precise, Nature is abundant, she gives, she is creative, she is still a mystery. Nature simultaneously co-operates and competes, Nature shares and guards her resources, Nature has impeccable timing. A heart-centred approach to shinrin-yoku bridges the language barriers with love, and restores our sacred connection.[105]

The evidence supporting *shinrin-yoku*

The term *shinrin-yoku* literally means a forest bath or shower. It was first used in the current context by Mr Tomohide Akiyama, the former head of the Japanese Forestry Agency, in an article on the 'blueprint for the *shinrin-yoku*', in the *Asahi Shimbun* newspaper of 29 July 1982.[106] Akiyama's colleague Yoshi-fumi Miyazaki is now a retired university professor, researcher, and Deputy Director of the Center for Environmental Sciences at the University of Chiba.

Miyazaki had been approached by the Japanese government to come up with ways of addressing endemic stress-related health problems amongst Japan's working population. At the time, information was available about the volatile oils that trees emit, but measuring and gathering physiological information in the field was still in its infancy. After several successful 'informal' walks where anecdotal evidence for the efficacy of forest bathing was gathered, in 1990 Prof. Miyazaki collaborated with the Japanese broadcaster

NHK to film a *shinrin-yoku* study on Yakushima Island off the southern coast, home to some of the country's oldest and most pristine rainforest, with trees thought to be up to 5000 years old.

The research focused on demonstrating the physiological effects of relaxation by measuring decreased levels of the stress hormone cortisol in saliva. This documentary really put the practice of forest bathing on the map, and since then we have seen a rapid development in accurate field measuring tools and a broader interest in investigating various physiological impacts of forest bathing, in parallel with a growing understanding of the psychological effects and implications. There is now a burgeoning body of evidence collected both in the field and in clinical settings to support the use of *shinrin-yoku* as a bona fide pathway towards wellbeing.

Prof. Miyazaki would undoubtedly have taken inspiration from the traditional native religion of Shinto for ideas about people going on walks through forests; Japan has 68 per cent forest cover[107] – unique for such an industrialised and heavily populated country (the UK has only 13 per cent, the second lowest of major countries in Europe).[108] Most accessible forests in Japan that have escaped felling are sacred forests, and sacred forests generally have a Shinto shrine in them. All land adjacent to the shrine is considered sacred due to the presence of *kami* or spirits. Historically, Shinto devotees made lengthy pilgrimages to various Shinto shrines across the country to pray for healing and success and to honour the spirits of their ancestors.

The basis of *shinrin-yoku* was formed by bringing together aspects of this ancient animistic religion with the ancient forests, and the recent understanding of the influence of volatile oils given off by trees; add to this a basic understanding of our evolutionary history, and how we are hardwired and adapted for nature connection (*biophilia*), and we have a potent and cost-effective method to determine and prove that being in Nature is good for us.

A wealth of evidence and information is available in books and online research papers, but to summarise the main clinical findings so far, *shinrin-yoku* has been shown to:

- increase natural killer (NK) cell count within the body, which boosts the immune system

- increase anti-cancer proteins

- decrease stress markers like cortisol

- increase parasympathetic nervous system activity and decrease sympathetic nervous system activity

- improve sleep disorders

- improve negative mood states like depression and anxiety

- improve cardiovascular health and regulate blood pressure, heart rate variability, and pulse rate

- improve metabolic health and weight loss

- lower blood sugar levels

- improve concentration and memory

- improve energy

- inspire feelings of awe and appreciation.

Before we examine these findings in more detail, I should state that I do not know whether the health issues studied were chosen because of their population morbidity rates or because of funding interests, whether many health issues were investigated and these results reflect only the ones that responded most positively, or whether there were wider epidemiological factors involved.

I am interested in how the forest influences illness or pathology, and vice versa. It's also worth considering that perhaps these illnesses arose because we stopped frequenting and living in the forest in the first place. Disorders such as those listed above could be side-effects of being removed from the crucible of our being. The finely tuned human body is programmed for efficient survival in forest environments close to the equator in Africa, and from an evolutionary perspective, we have not evolved to cope with the onslaught of stimuli and microscopic pollution that we are now subjected to. It's the small invisible things that we can't see that destroy us, not the sabre-toothed tiger.

All of our bodies contain minute amounts of toxic heavy metals and 'forever' chemicals, pesticides, and new viruses; airborne pollution affects 99 per cent of the global population.[109] This chronic stream of airborne and other chemical pollutants has a slow, insidious effect on our overall health and immune function, as the body misinterprets micropollutants as bacteria, which causes inflammation throughout the body. Being in the forest and breathing in the forest air (tree pollen notwithstanding) has an instant impact of reversing so many of these toxins and imbalances; we know this from our studies of the composition of the forest air and our understanding of the properties of so many of the tree essential oils and terpenes.

Since the start of the Industrial Revolution, migration from rural to urban areas has increased dramatically: the World Economic Forum estimates that over 55 per cent of the world's population or 4.3 billion people live in cities, and that number is set to grow to an estimated 80 per cent by 2050.[110] Apart from the obvious need to create more green spaces in cities and urban planning, the need to get people from the cities back out into Nature becomes paramount. We also need to consider how that loss of cultural connection to the land will affect the health of future generations (and also the obvious question, 'If everyone is living in the city, who is out on the land growing our food?').

I believe we would benefit from adopting a model that sees us as an intrinsic part of the forest. Although we perceive ourselves as very separate from Nature, we are actually the forest extended into hominid form. Forest designed us and nurtured our physiological, anatomical, and psychological processes. We are an extension of forest consciousness and forest community, we have a niche within that web, so we experience a powerful shift when we return home to the forest; those healing processes were always a part of our biology and ecology, indispensable in many ways. Remember that no single organism in this world exists in isolation, from the macro to the quantum level.

> According to some, our minds deal with more stimuli in a day than primitive people faced in a year. This will have a considerable effect on a young developing mind – not all negative I'm sure, but I do wonder what happens to the developing neural pathways of young children's brains when they are exposed to so much external stimuli, particularly when they can't differentiate virtual reality from true reality.

Research by Prof. Miyazaki, Dr Qing Li, and others demonstrates statistical evidence that time spent in the forest improves health and is therefore beneficial to include in programmes of preventive medicine. Some baseline results from Miyazaki's meta study of 2014 indicate the following positive results compared to an urban control group[111]:

- 12.4% decrease in cortisol level

- 7.0% decrease in sympathetic nervous activity

- 1.4% decrease in systolic blood pressure

- 5.8% decrease in heart rate

- 55% enhanced parasympathetic nervous system (PNS) activity.

These figures clearly indicate a reduction in stress states as a result of exposure to the forest environment, and enhanced PNS activity indicates a relaxed and healing state. Experiments were conducted comparing sitting and walking groups, and results were very similar compared to the control groups. Also of primary interest are the effects of forest bathing on immune function in the optimisation of lymphocytes or specialist natural killer (NK) cells. These NK cells have the capacity to detect and eliminate cancer cells; it is suggested that one day of walking in the forest will elevate NK cell counts for up to one month afterwards:

> Li *et al.* demonstrated that immune function was enhanced by forest therapy in middle-aged employees who volunteered to participate in these experiments. Natural killer cell activity, an indicator of immune function, was enhanced by 56% on the second day and returned to normal levels. A significant increase of 23% was maintained for 1 month even after returning to urban life, clearly illustrating the preventive benefits of forest therapy.[112]

Dr Li also conducted experiments which showed a forest bathing walk improved the quantity and quality of sleep by 15 per cent. In an interview, Dr Li, he stated that his team could only reproduce 50 per cent of the effects of the forest artificially through air diffusion of hinoki oils and by participants viewing forest landscapes, and said the other 50 per cent was due to the mystery of the forest. It seems that it is our immersion in the forest environment and its impact on all our senses and our ecology that is a vital aspect of the health and healing process. We cannot isolate and reduce these effects down and synthesise them, as has been happening recently with psychedelics.

Forest therapy/medicine seeks to establish itself as a legitimate intervention within applied medical science by being completely evidence based. I agree with the premise of this *and* the need to factor in the total homogenising effects of the forest environment. The empirical evidence across spans of time and the beauty and comfort these places offer us can sometimes be unquantifiable in words or statistics, because they speak to the spirit.

The power of *shinrin-yoku*

I have witnessed many remarkable transformations of people's lives through *shinrin-yoku* practices. It is impossible to pinpoint any particular reason why this happens, other than it feels like an organic catalyst for a change where a person was floundering, either due to stress, workload, life demands, or illness, or was feeling adrift in life or directionless. I believe that these transformations are partly due to accessing a wild, vestigial survival mechanism (see Chapter 13, The Savage Self, for more details). It is also because Nature seems to sweep through us, clearing out the dross and washing it downstream to be recycled. We are often left with a renewed feeling of expansion, a shift in perspective, and greater sense of altruism or virtue.

Being in the forest and the totality of forest environments somehow act as a complex adaptogen (a type of plant that has the capacity to regulate physiological processes and return the person to homeostasis). Certain herbs have the capacity to adapt their agency to excite us if we are low in energy, and calm us if we are overstimulated. The forest seems to provide what we need, or perhaps we are subconsciously drawn to what we need within the forest experience.

Over many years of working with clients, I've noticed this catalytic effect happen when the person is ready, as if Nature doesn't give us more than we can cope with at any time, and this for me is an important aspect of the therapeutic process – that we can trust that an individual will receive something of benefit in their growth journey at the point when they are open to fully receiving it. Patience, understanding, and trust are key in this process, to allow what is happening to naturally unfurl and reveal itself before us.

The walk leader cultivates an unconditional, nonjudgemental approach to a client's perspectives and towards specific locations. We have to develop trust in Nature's wisdom through observing it within ourselves. In our own personal practice and intimate relationship with Nature, and by thinking in longer time spans than the bitesize chunks of our staccato lives, we need to watch Nature flow, and step back from any desire to tinker or intervene. The main therapeutic power of *shinrin-yoku* walks is the slowing down. If we engaged the senses at our usual busy speed, we would become overstimulated or we would miss the deeper entry points into conscious connection. Slowing down creates space for reflection and for autonomic regulation.

I have created four basic principles of Nature Connection. They may seem to resemble descriptions of mindfulness practices, but they are distinct and have a subtly different orientation:

- Slow down.

- Notice.

- Be mindless.

- Reciprocate.

When we take each of these in turn, we begin to build our connection, establish our strong core, and feel the energy of our reaffiliation with Nature.

Slowing down

I need silence like I need air. I need to give my system time and space to be still and to process all the events that occur in daily life. Slowing down sounds like such a simple and easy thing to do, but should not be underestimated as the primary route towards wellbeing. Our bodies have a natural rhythm just as the Earth does, and by slowing everything down, by moving slowly through the forest, so much tension simply falls away; we become in sync with those ecological rhythms of forest life. My Buddhist friend Duncan says his meditation teacher speaks about being 'perky' – being in a relaxed but alert state, a bit like a cat or wild animal.

Slowing down affords us the opportunity to recalibrate our internal systems, particularly the brain and nervous system. Most of our physiological and some of our psychological processes work on feedback loops. Chemical (hormonal) and neural messengers relay information to the brain which then initiates actions to bring the body back into homeostasis; once the issue is resolved, signals are sent to the brain to cease that action and switch off the response. This is particularly true of our endocrine system which is involved in controlling our moods, and our adrenal and cortisol responses to threat and stress.

When walking slowly through the woods, our sensory inputs send a strong message to the brain that we are safe, and so the fight or flight response can be switched off. The constant internal babble which mirrors the constant stream of daily distractions quietens down, and we can relax. This leads to an increase in PNS activity, helping us to rest, relax, digest, and heal, and so reach a more optimum level of functioning. Other factors, such as the effects of the phytoncides, the restorative environment, the fascination, and the effects of shifting focus, also have important roles to play in our physiological response, in addition to the breath (which I will address separately).

Another key consideration is the environment itself and the quality of energy in that locale. Factors such as weather, light, temperature and appropriate clothing, composition and size of area, proximity to traffic noise, sight of buildings, litter, and other human traffic in the woods can have a significant influence on engagement (places with no other human contact are best for maximum effects). Some of these factors have been investigated by Kaplan and Kaplan in a concept called Attention Restoration Theory (ART), that attempts to define which particular components of the natural environment are the most effective for restoring a sense of wellbeing.[113]

Our *shinrin-yoku* participants often declare that although they have walked through a particular area of woodland all their lives, they had never really noticed it before in this new way, and now they are seeing it again as if for the first time with fresh eyes. They also say that they can never go back to seeing it how it was before, and that they will come back and forest bathe on a regular basis. This is partly due to them bringing a conscious focus to being present within the woods. This is facilitated by slowing down, leaving the dog behind, switching off the mobile phone, and refraining from chatting for the duration of the visit. The fact that they have been coming to these particular woods for so long indicates that there is something important and nurturing about this place for them (or perhaps they are just convenient of course!).

Every forest is different, with a different personality and zones of influence within it. Participants, if allowed to roam free, may be unconsciously drawn towards particular parts of the forest that we as practitioners may seek to avoid, judging them to be somehow undesirable. This is worth noting and interrogating to understand what this area signifies for us, what threat it holds, or how we feel about this corner of the woods. It is important for us as practitioners to be aware of our biases and be curious about places we subconsciously avoid in the woods, and places we are drawn to. It is desirable to move towards a curious, non-judgemental acceptance of all zones of the forest for our own personal development, and on behalf of our clients' needs. (See Chapter 8, Into the Forest, where I further explore how to perceive and work collaboratively with the different energies of the forest, and how this affects our therapeutic work with groups and also with one-to-one clients.)

One final image that comes to mind when I think of the power of shifting to slow time comes from Bruce Chatwin's excellent book *The Songlines*. Chatwin recounts being driven across the Australian desert in a truck with his fellow passenger, an Aboriginal man called Limpy. They are tracing Limpy's songlines, ancestral energy lines in the landscape that hold the songs of the stories of the land and his particular clan. At a certain point, they enter a gulley and Limpy starts babbling incoherently. They have to stop the vehicle because they realise that the songlines have to be sung at walking pace, and the truck was going too fast for Limpy to sing all the features of the land within the song. It strikes me that this is the same for all of us – when we slowly traverse the living Earth, we can begin to hear the songs of the ancestors and the land once more.

Walking speed

There are five walking speeds, although they may not always be distinct in our forest bathing sessions.

- Running: this is more of an advanced technique and will not be discussed here, but there is a place for running in our repertoire within very specific circumstances.

- Normal walking pace: we might utilise this as we walk from one gathering place to another, or on our way back after the session if it closes in the forest. It's nice for people who have been focused for a length of time to step out of that place and chat with each other at the end of the session if they want to. It can lead to some good outcomes, as can walking back in silence. Normal walking pace is also deployed as required in other situations.

- Slow walking pace: this is where we start to pay greater attention to what's around us and within us, and the awe and wonder of the woods takes effect. Simply walking slowly seems to engender silence, and calm descends on the group. I think this slow walking can also resemble stalking prey, hence the sensory enhancement.

- The really slow pace: it is important to differentiate this ultra slow pace from the regular slow pace as it adds another dimension to the work. The really slow pace happens when we ask participants to be moved by the forest, so that instead of initiating our own impulse to move, we wait until the moment when we are compelled forward (or any other direction) by the breath of the forest, the sky, or the waves. It is about returning to that gentle rhythm of life, that passive momentum. (See the exercise in the box below.)

- No movement or walking at all: however, within this poised state there is the origin of movement, slight energetic adjustments. Travel that is nuanced, graceful, and from within stillness; just like the midwinter forest, everything asleep and silent yet also moving down below and within, generating power from the still core, from the roots.

Ultra slow pace exercise

After some preliminary walking at the slow pace, perhaps in silence, and once in the middle of the forest, we can stop, perhaps taking off our footwear if desired. The instruction then is to stand still with eyes open or closed and simply wait for our bodies to be drawn in a particular direction. We feel the connection to the Earth, we may feel a pulse within us, and we wait until we lean in a particular direction. Imagine that you have a thin gossamer thread attached to your heart, and Nature is on the other end of that thread pulling you so gently, beckoning, weaving you into the fabric of the woods. If you resist, you can snap the thread; if you surge forward, you lose the gentle tension that guides you hither and thither.

You don't know where you are going, or where you will end up; ego is having a nap. Your movements are almost imperceptible, and your body is moving with the shapes around you, mirroring the slow trees, the dripping moss, the rotting leaves, the creatures of the forest floor, and the breeze on your face. Your breath moves in and out like the surge of the tide, waiting for the forest to pull you forward on the breath, and then stopping, waiting, and moving again. A pulse. Take your time; there is no rush, no need to be anywhere or go anywhere, just a total surrender. If you wind up in a spot that feels right, just stop there a while, slow, slow movements, no thoughts, just somatic awareness in space.

Allow plenty of time for this exercise and don't put a time limit on it, but suggest an approximation, say 30 minutes. Establish a meeting point prior to the exercise, and conduct the exercise in an area with some naturally defined boundaries – otherwise, people will be gone forever!

Noticing

Of course, when we slow down, we then begin to notice things, things that we would have ordinarily missed completely. More subtle things now catch our eye; we prick up our ears, sniff a good scent, brush against a wet leaf. We are receding back or growing into our primitive sharp faculties, and our awakening senses are picking up these previously imperceptible details and intelligences. What do we notice, what are we drawn to investigate? I love watching gnats on the evening air in a spot where the sun slants down on to the river surface; they are such fascinating creatures and seem to be having a big gnat speed dating get-together. I would never notice that detail of life in my ordinary 'getting on with stuff' mode, and yet when I watch these little beings who only live for a week, my soul is uplifted, I feel spacious and free, and tearful as I ponder the exquisite animate life in everything.

Our participants start to notice what is all around them, particularly in the micro-realms of the mini beasts, the moss forests, the lichens, the flower buds, and the playful delicate patterns in so many things, and then look up and take in the vast cathedral of the canopy, and the sky beyond, the falling raindrops, the swirling tree tops in the wind – this is the total immersion. Simply by noticing all these stimuli, this suffusion of organic beauty bathing our fragile being with love, there is no sense of the self as other in this ego-disintegration process.

A 10x magnifying hand lens (sometimes referred to as a Ruper or loupe lens) is a great tool for this deeper observing process, bringing us up close to the mini forest worlds (and when I bring my focus down so small, I feel conversely like I'm suddenly connected to the vast cosmos).

Noticing is not just about what we can see; it's about the whole panoply of sensuous exchange, external and internal sensations and movements (see Chapter 10, The Senses, for more detail on how each of our senses are brought into experiential enquiry and interplay). Noticing is also when we can begin to hear the stories from deep within the Earth, and from these stories myths and songs emerge, and from our deep noticing we are informed about life, just like the Taoists, the ancient Greeks, and in the oral traditions of Indigenous Peoples.

We have to slow down to take in the character and depths of our plant and animal cousins; their evolved ways of being in the world have so much to teach us, as we are a conglomerate of evolutionary experiences and trials. When we sense another creature's or plant's energy, we notice that resonance, that kinship within us; we don't need to actively do anything, simply notice, observe, and our psyche then translates or filters it, and we may experience an ontological shift in some part of our selves, or we may feel less constricted.

When we go slowly and gently, the song of the land beneath us itself invites our full embodied presence to hear those resonant notes; every part of Nature has a voice for us.

Mindlessness

Mindlessness is about taking the locus of our self from the mind into the body and the bodymind – animal mind. Mindfulness meditation has become increasingly popular in mainstream Western culture over the last 20 years, partly due to the efforts of many meditation teachers, and scientific research-ers like Jon Kabat-Zinn, professor of medicine and stress reduction, who describes mindfulness as our capacity for awareness and self-knowing.[114] Mindfulness can be cultivated by paying attention, and Kabat-Zinn further describes it as being nothing out of the ordinary, nothing particularly special, although utterly transformative for both the individual and collective.

Mindfulness is being in a state of noticing what is present without judging it, and this non-judging is an important aspect of the forest bathing experi-ence too. We are constantly judging things in everyday life, compelled by our preferences and prejudices. Somehow coming out into the woods allows us to drop all of that pressure; the mind has nothing to fight against or to try to socially measure itself by. The canopy above us and the multisensory input have a disarming effect, as does standing looking at the sea and the sky.

The question which arises is that if we are not paying attention, not being aware in the present, then where are we? Surely, surely present time awareness and being attentive to our surroundings is our default position in life. I'm keen to know where people are if they are not present, where have they gone. I know that I can be a bit dreamy at times, but my dreaming is in Nature or with Nature – not always, I admit. There are plenty of times when I haven't had enough sleep, or I'm a bit stressed and then I am a little pre-occupied, but I have managed to cross the road safely so far. Maybe it helps that I have spent some considerable time being hyper-vigilant, but I tend to notice everything, every detail, every person walking past me, every driver, details of places and the people in them – it's exhausting! So when I come out into the woods or go down and swim in my beautiful local river the Dart, which runs through the woods here on the edge of the moor, I just come into peace, silence, no thoughts at all, just a kind of neutral or filled up with non-intrusive sensory stimuli place. A place of expansive, tranquil liberation, a place of empty mind or mindlessness.

About 15 years ago, I had an epiphany moment in realising that my life wasn't flowing. There was so much energy going into everything, and so little reward, I kept feeling thwarted, or blocked. Establishing Ecotherapy as a legitimate healing modality led me to many closed doors and indifference. I realised that my attempts were not bearing fruit, and so I decided to stop paying attention to my mind, my constant ruminations, those voices of self-doubt, sabotage, and the old inner critic. I did this by deciding to listen to what my body was telling me, to focus on just a somatic wisdom way of relating to the world, and this re-prioritising actually took me back to a child-like acceptance and playfulness, and into unbounded creativity. It might seem irresponsible or vague, but it wasn't at all – it was an act of kindness to self, to just listen to the body's voice and gently shift priorities; it was very helpful and grounding.

So mindlessness doesn't mean gratuitous violence and indiscriminate vandalism; it simply refers to this sense of allowing the body to lead and putting the mind back in its place – as servant and not as master. The mind is just a useful tool to bring out of its box occasionally to solve a problem or bolster an intellectual debate on some topic, but otherwise, and definitely out in Nature, it goes back on the lead and waits to be called. Our bodies have primacy out here, and our body minds tell us all we need to know. Just watch people walking through the woods talking – the minds are engaged and they are not in the same woods that you are in, sitting silently under a tree.

Becoming mindless can either be cultivated or can happen spontaneously just like being mindful, and their qualities are related. I spoke with my colleague Duncan Moss, a Buddhist and mindfulness teacher, about these comparisons:

Me: Where does mindfulness come from?

D: Mindfulness comes from human beings. And as much as I think it's been here since the dawn of time, since people became aware that they had a mind, the actual word mindfulness does have strong links with Buddhist teachings. I think it's a much broader tradition than Buddhism.

Me: So, the link with Buddhism and Buddhist teachings that you mentioned, is that a particular teaching of the Buddha or is there a tradition that it comes from?

D: One of the Buddha's early teachings was called Four Foundations of Mindfulness: mindfulness of body, mindfulness of feelings, mindfulness of mind, and mindfulness of Dhamma. As we know, language and translation are tricky things. The Buddha was teaching in Pali, and then later Buddhism was translated into Sanskrit, Tibetan, etc., so the modern English word mindfulness is obviously a translation. You can argue that there is definitely a stream of teachings from the Buddha through to later writers and teachers in Buddhism, to the kind of modern mindfulness, the use of that word.

Me: One of the things that I teach is mindlessness, which is very different from mindfulness. I'm trying to encourage people to get away from the mind, out of the mind, and just be completely focused in the body, which is in contrast to mindfulness. But what is the desired outcome of mindfulness?

D: To go back what you were saying about mindlessness, as I understand it, what you're describing is another form of mindfulness because, of course, you've got the loaded language with the word *mind* in the word mindfulness.

Effectively, the Buddhist teachings describe heartfulness, not mindfulness, so they are more about being rooted in the heart. The Tibetan tradition says that all mindfulness and meditation practices are about awareness, and awareness is not just a mind thing in terms of our brains. It's also about the body, our whole body is a tool of awareness – our heart and guts and all the senses are tools of awareness. So, if heartfulness is embodied awareness, the mind is then just the mind as we know it, which is those chattering bits that we associate with the brain.

Duncan's description puts me in mind of the Tantric traditions that were a part of certain Hindu and Buddhist scriptures, prior to some of these practices becoming Westernised. Tantra is considered as distinct from many other spiritual traditions in that the focus is on liberation through the physical body rather than via transcendence of it. Through breath and other specific exercises, Tantric practices are established to direct universal energies into the practitioner as a means of breaking free from ignorance and suffering. In contrast to many ascensionist religious practices, where the focus is on sending energy upwards either from the heart or the head towards a heaven or deity, Tantra is largely about an embodied awareness which includes the heart, guts, and genitals as part of the 'descentionist' route through the body to the Earth, to enable union with the Divine.

Of course, this is exactly what we are seeking through our forest bathing practice, to become so fully embodied that we feel truly alive, animated, and aware; we are alert, yet relaxed, in tune with our surroundings, as if we were an intrinsic part of this landscape, this ecology, this forest home. The sensory awareness exercises are a fundamental part of this process, but must not be mistaken for the purpose or goal of forest bathing; they are simply a vector for entry to a deeper level of awareness, in the bodily felt equivalent of meditation or Tantric practice. The mind becomes absorbed (and therefore childlike and non-encroaching) through the embodied and novel curious exploration of our natural world.

This mindlessness is a liberation from the constraints of dogma, and the rationalising (fearful) non-stop thinking. In order to fully give participants the subconsciously conveyed permission to enter this mindless space, we as walk leaders must be strong, confident, and calm. We must embody that holding and containment that people need in order to feel safe and let go. We must also be comfortable with our own vulnerability; our own sadness or grief may arise in the forest, and be present in our circle.

People are desperately seeking authenticity and connection, and so we must make sure we can offer these with reassurance and careful, sensitive facilitation; we are simultaneously holding a person or group, and holding all of the Nature energy and communication too.

Reciprocity

The fourth and perhaps the most important aspect of Nature connection is how we can give back – how to feel a sense of reciprocity with Nature when we are in the woods (see Chapter 7 for a fuller discussion).

Reciprocity emerges from an appreciation of systems theory, which states that we cannot understand a living system in isolation, and that in order to understand the properties of each of its parts, we need to understand the organisation of the whole; we need to look at ecological communities and understand the subtle mutual relationships between each organism within it.

For example, when I was devising a forest bathing programme for primary schools, I realised one of the key learnings was that everything in Nature completes a circle or a cycle. Everything returns to the beginning; there is no waste or surplus within the system, and yet Nature creates an abundant harvest where she can. An oak tree only needs one acorn to germinate and grow for it to have passed on its DNA to its progeny, so why are there more acorns than required to repopulate or occupy that ground? Why are some years 'mast' years with a bumper crop of seeds and nuts and berries? By the time the next spring comes around, everything is returning back to the earth and the cycle starts again. What was not eaten, or germinated into a new plant, has become rich humus and mulch for the next crop, all nutrients being recycled. Somehow I needed to incorporate this basic premise of self-sustainability.

There is no sense of self-sustaining equilibrium within capitalist ideology; a culture that promotes infinite growth within a closed resource system can never be sustainable. Capitalism is an abstraction of reason; it is outside the realms of Nature and natural law. Looking at all of the incredible, complex feedback loop systems and how they all work together felt like the best way of demonstrating both homeostasis and autopoiesis for the school programme.

When we develop an understanding of ecological communities, we can appreciate that living systems are part of a greater web of life. This web of life consists of networks within networks.[115] Ultimately, we return to the bare facts of our interdependence within these ecosystem networks. We are an organism with networks and communities existing within us; we are a part of a larger biosphere, and the Earth itself, although a closed self-sustaining system, is dependent on the Sun, without which it would be a lifeless hunk of rock floating in space. Our solar system is itself part of a larger galaxy, and so on, with everything connected.

We may feel disempowered to make change in this world, but a conscious acknowledgement of reciprocity is the antidote to this, because it shifts the zeitgeist away from toxic exploitation, and towards ecological cycle living. Yes, it is important that we fly less, consume less, drive less, recycle as much as possible, and shop and vote ethically – all of that is critical – but personal reciprocity gives us the power to change.

What that may look like on the ground with our groups is to offer something back as an energetic exchange. If we sense that simply turning up is enough, then it is; but if we can offer a gift in exchange for what we have received over the last 10 million years, then that is also good. Some suggestions are poems, songs, prayers, pieces we have written, dances and movements with the trees and soil, and food and drinks. Make a meal for the forest spirits and come out and share it with the trees; drinks and libations are also good at propitious times of year. Please don't bring unsightly offerings or altars to the woods; when you leave, there must be no sign that you have been there, so if you do build an altar, and bring fruit and flowers, for example, please keep it discreet and sensitive to others. Take home any non-organic items and clean up before you leave, say thanks, and enjoy the sharing. (See also 'Reciprocity' in Chapter 7.)

Another way of offering something back to the forest, which can be done with selective discernment, is to offer any of your bodily fluids to the Earth and the trees. Done with intention, this is a powerful, magical, and metaphorical way of mutual exchange with the forest. Perhaps ask the forest before you discharge yourself in the woods!

We can also offer our feelings to the trees. Some may consider this abusive, but the trees have been here a lot longer than us and they are generally happy to receive our feelings. Once again, I suggest you gently check in with the trees first. We can offer our sadness and rage, jealousy, grief, depression, fury, and confusion; they all are welcome and they become composted down, part of the rich humus layer to form food and nutrients for the growing roots and seeds of new life.

If you wish to start a new creative endeavour or a new life for yourself, one of the ways in which you can share this with the woods is to go out for the day and find the right place in the woods where you feel safe and relaxed. Spend some time with the trees there, maybe one in particular you feel called to. Establish a dialogue, tell the tree your ideas and dreams, and if the moment feels right, dig down through the leaf mulch and gather a small pinch of the rich black soil. Smell it up close; it is sweet and full of life (one gram of soil can contain as many as 50 billion bacteria). Now form the soil into a shape whilst offering your intentions. If you want, you can add a small amount of spit to the mix and mould the soil before reburying it deep within the blanket of rotting leaves. Many of the creation myths and other stories from around the world incorporate this idea of a god or goddess or mortal mixing some spit with clay or earth to create new life. Give huge thanks and love and pass on your way; your ideas are gestating in the warmth of the ground, nurtured by the tree guardians.

Relationship, Reciprocity, The Dance

We are witnessing incontrovertible evidence of climate change and planetary heating. More extremes of temperature and weather events, records being broken for heat, wind, rain, etc. This is just the beginning of the final chapter, whilst, somewhat uncomprehendingly, politicians are urging more growth. Is that a disconnect, or a deception? I don't know what the whole solution is – I don't think anyone does, or is courageous enough to take action – I just know it can't go on like this. It is unsustainable; we can't go on taking and not giving, as is the same with any personal relationship. The problem is not only with what we are doing, but also with what we are not doing.

We seem to have lost our capacity to be reverential as part of sensitivity, to be moved to change our consumer patterns and experience having fewer personal belongings (i.e., stuff) and more personal belonging in our world which provokes pro-environmental behaviours. Beneath the carapace of indifference, we yearn for that contact with the wild animal in our lives; maybe at a subconscious level we realise our kinship, and just as it's too late, we gaze longingly out at our cousins in the woods simultaneously yearning for their acknowledgement and love, whilst knowing that we are unwittingly destroying our own salvation with theirs.

Maybe that is one of the lessons of this time, that money and status won't protect you from viruses, and that connection to others is more important than material things, or to live each day as if it's your last. That is my hope for the topics raised by this book: to nurture a respect for Nature and our personal psychotherapy that occurs in direct contact with the natural world. Healing is mutual. Remember Mary Oliver's advice in 'Wild Geese': 'You only have to let the soft animal of your body love what it loves.' And yet, how hard is it for us to be that animal, to embody our animal ancestry and to move from that core within, yielding to the environment around us seamlessly, and with kind compassion?

Sometimes I observe that we have lost a loving gentle connection to our bodies. It's a complex topic influenced by cultural pressures, but how often are we either lazy and detached from the idea that we inhabit a body, or take them to the gym and flog them, or go running with an app, but is that a connection or another enslavement? How mindful is that? Are we really leaning into the voice of our body? Connecting with our bodies means connecting with the sacred, connecting with what is gently heroic within us, or just listening in to the messages our bodies give us, before they start shouting at us which is normally just before we enter A&E. In Nature, we are embodied; it may take time to get there, but we can find that connection.

Our lives have become homogenised into something without edges, without peaks, and without the depths of appreciation that come from an embodied, hard, yet well-lived life. We were designed to burn the candle brightly, to taste the true vitality of existence, to look up, TO LOOK UP!, to see the sky and wonder, to see the stars and feel our place within all that is. (Can you see the sky right now as you read this?)

Most of us defer true joy, defer true connection. To allow the opening of self to self and self to other than self remains problematic. If I open up to the mysteries of the Universe, how will I ever get myself back into the box? If my heart opens, and I am vulnerable and I fully breathe, who might I be then? That time in Nature is a subversive encouragement to be authentic, be animal and embodied. What if I became my own hero, if I committed to heroic deeds, being true to myself and taking that brave decision to quit my job, and go back to drama school, law school, clown school, mountaineer school, or whatever that thing was that we dreamed of as young innocents, but were prevented from exploring because of disapproval or other constraints? What then? As Mary Oliver asks us:

Tell me, what is it you plan to do with your one wild and precious life?[116]

If we can't just take off and live in the hills or sail the seas, then we can develop meaningful associations with Nature closer to home in our daily lives. A local wood might not seem so dramatic, but it is quality not quantity that makes the difference, and that's where the deeper realms of *shinrin-yoku* come in. Simply by slowing the pace, embracing the animal body – the Savage Self – and allowing our awareness and curiosity to emerge from the shell, we can have these elevated states of transdimensional consciousness and mini-epiphanies.

By visiting a place on a regular basis, we witness the miracle of the seasons unfolding before us and it calms and reassures us, gives us hope, or perspective, or balance, or realisation. All we need to do is just show up. There are whole mini-worlds to explore in a clump of mosses and liverworts growing out of a stone wall: the scurrying of the woodlouse and the delicate threads of the spider's web. I can lose myself for hours watching the birds in my back garden, and studying their behaviour feels like the Universe revealing itself through their motions and vivid rainforest colours. I feel that I am a part of this participatory Universe, part of that exquisite sensual dance: co-mingling energy responding to my partner's movements and expressing my own in a symbiotic exchange.

> At the still point of the turning world. Neither flesh nor fleshless;
> Neither from nor towards; at the still point, there the dance is,
> But neither arrest nor movement. And do not call it fixity,
> Where past and future are gathered. Neither movement from nor
>   towards,
> Neither ascent nor decline. Except for the point, the still point,
> There would be no dance, and there is only the dance.[117]

It's this reciprocal exchange that brings balance to the Universe, harmony to the life forms and joy felt within. Are we the only creatures that can appreciate beauty? I'm not so sure that just because we have a particular expression of consciousness, we alone can experience aspects of self-realisation – birds play on thermals just for the joy of it, dolphins surf the bow wave...

A recurring theme in these chapters is relationship, being in right relationship with the land and with all manifestations of life, human and non-human. Reciprocating and exchanging gifts with Nature and altruistic acts help to forge a lifetime of security and calmness within. Being grounded in the perpetual flow, we finally come home to truth and that eudaemonic happiness, and hopefully we don't fall into the trap of taking ourselves too seriously.

CHAPTER 7

Health

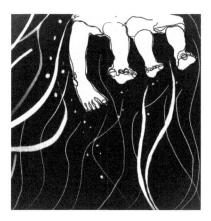

'The Earth is our Mother.' This has become an overused, trite slogan commonly associated with a certain hippy element of environmentalism, but as with so many truths that have since become clichés, it is worth remembering the veracity of the meaning.

The Earth is indeed our mother,[118] and there is an argument for a scientific, evidence-based statement to support this which I propose needs to be at the core of all of our decisions and endeavours, both personal and political, and adopted by global organisations like the United Nations. Let us examine this in more detail.

Disrespect for Nature

Looking around at this beautiful world, it is evident that we are not respecting our mother at all. Since the Agricultural and Industrial Revolutions, we have shaved off her hair (forests) and sliced open her skin (soil), mined deep inside her body to cut out her bones (minerals) and drain her blood (crude oil), poisoned her arteries and polluted her lungs, then filled her wounds with our toxic waste.

What kind of different society can we imagine where we treat our relationship to this 'Mother Earth' as sacrosanct, as our primary intercourse. We could put Nature first and love that which gives birth to us. What would that society or world look like to you? What sacrifices of comfort and technology would we have to forego in order to be in total harmony with this beautiful, fragile, dynamic biosphere, this expression of creative joy made manifest in self-sustaining form?

Only a very disturbed child would seek to abuse its mother in the way in which we treat our place in the Universe. What has happened for us to behave in this extraordinary manner, especially as we are so dependent on Earth for food, water, and breath? There is no other place to go, no other planet to move to and destroy after this one is finally sucked dry. There are other examples from the natural world where the organism destroys its host or environment, but these are rare exceptions and the organism has developed a way for its genetic material to survive.

How can we put our name to this madness? As a global community, we have become dominated by Western materialist values, supported by a 'science as religion' attitude, and in the same way in which *Homo sapiens* gradually muscled out other hominid species, so we are now in a second wave which seeks to eradicate all other cultural variations to achieve universal homogeneity, ubiquity, and total control. Yet although we are the dominant force and narrative at this time, we are certainly not the wisest. In a wonderful twist of irony, we call ourselves *Homo sapiens* which means 'the wise ones', but the title of 'wise one' was once reserved for those who knew about birth, health, and death, the healing powers of the land, and the plants and animals that we share a common language with.[119]

Fostering respect for the land

There is a plethora of scientific evidence and clinical studies to back up our understanding of how Nature can support a person's wellbeing. Unfortunately, from my perspective there are three obvious omissions or oversights from the Japanese clinical studies and those from around the globe associated loosely with eco-therapeutic or wilderness-type interventions and *shinrin-yoku*.

1. Reciprocity. There is no mention of the need or desire to offer back to Nature to ensure longevity and **sustainability**: in other words, if

we carried on this practice for another thousand years, how would it impact the planet? Where is our environmental impact assessment for this length of time?

2. Integrated self-care. If *shinrin-yoku* is designated as a form of health-care, how does that sit with how participants may lead other areas of their lives? Is it enough to just go for an occasional walk in the woods and then carry on as before? **Resilience**.

3. How are we honouring the indigenous practices and the unique ecologies of the areas that we operate in? How are we appropriating or diluting local customs and rituals? What language are we using that reinforces these practices (e.g., such terms as **sit-spot**)?[120]

Are we continuing to hurt ourselves and our planet?

It might come across as sanctimonious or even sentimentalist to suggest that we start to give something back to Nature; it might seem unscientific in some embarrassing way. Of course, in the West we don't have a full comprehension of the traditional Japanese cultural relationship to their forests, most of which have been preserved due to their Shinto shrines which give them protected sacred land status (see Chapter 5, Oriental Philosophy). We have a very different relationship with the environment in Europe and North America. Indeed, every country will have its own unique set of myths, stories, and cultural associations relating to the land, from which arise our political and environmental positions and discourses.

Our psychological traits also play an enormous part in the way that we interact with our environment, and those traits, whilst sharing some common variants, may also have regional and national differences. I notice in Europe a different attitude in relating to the environment which emanates from the love of food, wine, and the land – the 'terroir' (I love that word, you can taste the earth in that word, smell the wet soil). Europe and most of the US has lower population densities than here in the UK, and in Europe there are some better forestry management policies and hunting practices. Many people who live in the cities of Europe have a little cabin somewhere out in the woods, down by the shore, or up in the hills where the whole family can decamp in the summer months. This seems like a very civilised compromise, and I definitely feel there's more respect for Nature, but this also sits alongside conurbations of heavy industry and pollution.

Reciprocity

We cannot keep on taking and not giving back to the system which sustains us. In any form of Nature-based therapy, if what we are doing is to be sustainable and not just another on-trend distraction, then we have to incorporate an attitude of reciprocity in all we do within our own practice and also with our clients in Nature, otherwise our activities are akin to all the mining, quarrying, extracting, fracking, deforesting, drilling, and dumping that is going on each day. Regarding Nature as just a convenient resource or a free room for us to work in places us alongside those who exploit the earth for profit. Therapists have a responsibility to give back to the land that they use for their practices.

Right from the start, we can adopt a way of thinking, talking, and being that creates a balance between what we receive with what we can give, what the client can give back in return for holding, breathing, revelation, resolution, or succour. We create an energetic dance, a yin-yang dynamic; we may even be able to give back more than we took. How can we do this?

On a global scale, the human part of the problem is made up of people just like you and me, individuals all struggling to do their best, with immense moral and ethical dilemmas. We convert/cajole/persuade/entreat/enlist people to start treating the Earth with kindness one by one, one person at a time. Each human being counts, trust me. If that sounds evangelical, it's because I love my world and it's getting serious now – we're running out of time.

At an individual scale, we give back by learning partly from the wisdom of various indigenous peoples who have lived in harmony with their environment for hundreds or thousands of years – if they hadn't done so, they would no longer be here. Some civilisations have disappeared because they got too big, too hierarchical, too arrogant, and over-exploited the land, leaving them unable to respond to changes in Nature and fluctuating patterns of weather events like El Niño.

Indigenous tribal cultures around the globe acknowledge that delicate balance of life between themselves as apex predators and the ecological network that surrounds them and supports their existence. We have survived and thrived due to our resilience and adaptability, but wherever you go, you will meet local people who still revere the forces that can affect their lives. If they have a successful hunt, they offer some of their food back to the forest and give thanks to the spirit of the animal that offered its life for them. Sacrifice requires thanks and sacrifice in return. What can we sacrifice for what we receive from the Earth? Let's start thinking, acting, and praying differently; let's not assume that we have so much freedom anymore, that we are entitled to do what we damn well please.

We can all do the good work with recycling, refusing plastics, installing better insulation, consuming less, buying local, walking and cycling more, joining conservation groups, and lobbying for changes to environmental laws and protections for the land, and Earth jurisprudence. All of these are human-centred activities, and aim to restrict our footprint, not just carbon, but our ecological 'noise', and protect Nature which has no voice in the corporate board room (although local and regional governments are starting to listen to calls for personhood and citizenship rights to be acknowledged in law for rivers, forests, and mountains).[121]

Specifically, we give back when we make a personal sacrifice towards the land, we honour the elements and the seasons, we honour the wounds and we honour the tears, we repent, we rejoice, we supplicate, we process (as in procession), we make amends, we ask to rejoin the dance, we petition, we pray, and finally, most importantly, we reconcile! This is the single most important element of rebalancing the community and reducing climate change.

Ways to give back

What can we do? Just keep it simple, make an offering from the heart – please read Meister Eckhart's poem 'When I Was the Forest' in Chapter 13, The Savage Self. Bearing in mind that the poem was written in the 14th century (pre-Darwin), I believe Eckhart is saying that he remembers being each evolutionary stage and that they are a part of him, and he them, and is asking for their hand in marriage as a ritual, a blessing, a humbling of self, and a joining of forces.

Think of all the colourful, bizarre rites, ceremonies, celebrations, rituals, and festivities all over the world linked to the land and blessing the earth, fire, water, and sky. Create your own ritual, but keep it simple, light, fun, and sincere. There is much to be angry, sad, anxious, and solemn about, but by bringing our child-like attention to these rituals, we are not avoiding or denying the truths of these feelings; we are choosing to express our tenacious belief in Nature's way of bringing life on Earth back to homeostasis, and to joy.

Offer with good intentions any of your bodily fluids as a sacrifice for the land and the forest. Your tears of grief are the jewels of moisture transformed to joy and love by a tree's roots and the mycorrhizal systems under you – that's alchemy. Give away a part of yourself to feed the trees.

Give other offerings too. Sing a song. On one of my first training courses, a young woman had come all the way from the Czech Republic, and she went into the woods and sang a song that her mother had sung to her as a small child about home and the trees. I wept to hear its beauty, and also how the forest sighed with pleasure to receive such a treat. Usually, when we go to the woods, we walk around with our friends, mobile phones (!), or our dogs, and we never stop and say hello. The trees reach out their branches, so happy to see us, but we don't know how to stop and have a chat and a hug – we just get back in our cars and drive away – so when we offer a song or a dance or a prayer they are enraptured.

Poems and anything you have written will also go down well. Food, drink, libations, candles, incense, chocolate, cacao, nuts and seeds, drawings, and trinkets can all be offered. Just do it discreetly and respectfully. Attune yourself to what is appropriate and don't leave a mess for others. Use natural materials that will decay, don't leave non-biodegradable or gaudy things everywhere, and be sensitive.

In Cornwall at some of the sacred wells, there has long been a local tradition for tying a small piece of cloth from a sick person's garment to a branch of one of the trees next to the well or spring. These are called 'clarty rags' and the custom originates from the belief that the tree will suck out the illness from the rag, and that when the rag has rotted and fallen from the branch, the person is healed. Unfortunately, due to the huge increase in visitor numbers in recent years and a greater awareness of Cornwall's sacred sites, the trees are now smothered by all sorts of paraphernalia. It has become very unsightly and feels polluted; the place is drained of energy and is filled with sick people's hopes and needs (not their fault, and a reminder that we crave some real connection to the land).

Reconnection to Nature

It is important to step beyond the limitations of Western medicine with its mechanistic view of the body and reconnect ourselves to the body of the planet. We must move away from so many constrictive rules and regulations (notwithstanding the need to protect ourselves from litigation and from accidents), away from the refusal to acknowledge that there is a spiritual dimension to our lives. This is nothing to do with belief systems or gazing at sunsets and feeling awe; it's a basic component of how we are hardwired

– of how the spirit, the very essence of us, finds expression in the material dimension, and what that means for our spiritual evolution.

People are crying out for connection in response to the empty, vapid promises of power, status, and wealth. Forest bathing is an accessible and effective intervention to support people's health and encourage Nature-caring behaviours: 'Interventions designed to facilitate a stronger connection to nature may result in greater engagement in proenvironmental behavior... Nature connectedness is a strong psychological predictor of environmental concern and proenvironmental behaviors.'[122]

There is now an irrefutable body of evidence to support Nature connection as an efficacious intervention for wellbeing outcomes, and I hope that these findings will influence medical practitioners to recommend 'green prescriptions', either alongside or instead of mainstream medical interventions, particularly in the treatment of mild to moderate depression and anxiety.

Successful forest bathing interventions help individuals to interrogate their existing lives and discover lost or suppressed aspects of the psyche that contribute towards a more holistic or authentic way of living. A shift in perspective can establish a deeper appreciation for the natural world and its inhabitants, alongside fostering a more pro-social and pro-self-respecting approach to the body and mind. Anti-self behaviours such as alcohol consumption and over-eating can become less appealing after a meaningful encounter with Nature, and a conscious realisation or awakening to the voice of the body which by origin and association is also the voice of Nature external to the self.

Headmind versus bodymind

We come to conclusions and decisions about so many things on a daily basis, but how often do we question our decision-making processes? How many of those decisions are based on logic and how many on emotion? How did we arrive at that key moment in our lives and the direction it took us in? How many of us have made decisions we later regret with the benefit of hindsight? The truth is that we can never get it right all of the time, but hopefully as we age, we learn to develop greater scrutiny and perspicacity, and perhaps take more time in those processes to consider the effect on others.

We must also ask, who is making the decision? We all like to think that we are autonomous individuals with a will and a unique personality that guides us towards achieving more of what we want and less of what we find incompatible with our needs and values. It sounds simple and straightforward, but how often are our decisions truly our own? How often do we listen to the authentic voice within, or instead go with the flow, try to fit in, and not stir up the waters too much? We often bear witness to the upheaval and disturbance caused when a friend or family member suddenly makes a rash decision that sends ripples through that relational web.

The point here is that others are often invested in keeping us a particular way, in maintaining a status quo. Emotional Freedom Technique explains that when we were children, everybody else got to write on our 'wall of beliefs', except us. We grow up learning to make the decisions that others influence us to make, or alternatively rebelling and violently going in the other direction as a reaction.

Sometimes we also make decisions that go against who we really are, against our true nature. We do this when we either don't listen to the 'voice within' or we use our will and ego to override all subtle considerations. These are micro-aggressions against the self. This dichotomy occurs because we don't understand that our bodies have a mind and a voice, equally as valid as any dominant headmind thought processes. We rarely ever listen to the voice of the body, because we have been trained and programmed to ignore it, but the bodymind is our wise, protective, and instinctive character that emanates from survival needs.

About six years ago, I was facing a dilemma. I had two parallel careers, neither of which was particularly successful nor a failure, just sort of unsatisfactory. I remember one autumn day going for a walk with a good friend along the Brecon Canal in Wales. He said, 'Stefan, it's not possible to run two careers at the same time; you need to choose between them and just put your energy into making one successful.' Well, I wasn't having any of that! You see my two careers – my outdoor therapy work and my carpentry/design business – felt like the two arms of my body, I couldn't cut off one to grow the other, and I certainly couldn't choose which one to pursue and which to ditch. I wrestled with this conundrum for nearly a year.

My body and my head had two opposing viewpoints and the ongoing dialogue between them led to a stalemate. My body wanted the hard physical and technical aspects of the carpentry and design work, and my head wanted to return to full-time outdoor therapy work. My ego was striving for recognition in the design world, my heart was yearning for Nature; my caution was evident, and so I felt stuck in this impasse.

It was when I had an epiphany and put my bodyvoice first, and, significantly, prioritised creativity, that everything shifted in an instant. My body agreed that I could give up the carpentry and design work (which I considered a major part of my character as I perceived myself), and instead focus on developing the therapeutic Nature work, in exchange for taking up woodturning for pleasure so that I would still be engaged in working with wood and design, but crucially not for money. Once that opening had appeared and I was comfortable with it, the therapeutic Nature work took off; the phone started ringing and it hasn't stopped since.

The point of this anecdote is that it is always good to just sit with things and let them brew a little, and as I teach my students, just sit with the discomfort of not knowing something. Out of that chaos or directionless place emerges something new and profound. Prioritising my body and my soul immediately led to such a clear perspective; I have never felt happier in my life because I am working with my bodymind and not against it. My ego becomes more of the servant to my body/soul purpose, and I can just get on with things now feeling in greater alignment with my path. It sounds glib, but the qualitative difference is huge, and worth mentioning here. There are still challenges, but somehow, by feeling that I am on my path, I have this sense of ease.

Tuning in to the voice of the body is also part of Nature: it's no good setting out to be a *shinrin-yoku* practitioner or ecotherapist when you are out of touch with Nature, or actively going against your own nature, your own animal needs. Overriding this body or animal aspect of ourselves is not healthy and can lead to inner conflict, or thwarted plans, and ultimately illness.

We must be congruent between our bodies and our thoughts, but increasingly we ignore the fact that we are embodied creatures, that we have bodies that require our care – as one colleague puts it, the body just serves as a 'head taxi', getting us between the fridge and the sofa! Even great athletes may never listen in to the voice of the body, and simply override their body's warning signals with a strict training regime. This can frequently lead to illnesses like myalgic encephalomyelitis/chronic fatigue syndrome (ME/CFS).

Listening in to the body requires patience and sensitivity, awareness that we have a body, and that the body might have a slightly different agenda to us. We have to establish a dialogue, and when we take time out in Nature and walk slowly, it serves as an invitation to the body to let its voice become louder and be heard. Mary Oliver explains this beautifully in her poem 'Wild Geese' (see the full poem in Chapter 4). She offers, 'You only have to let the soft animal of your body love what it loves.' In other words, we can drop that Protestant work ethic lie and just let our soft animal selves do what they are made to do.

Health benefits of *shinrin-yoku*

You may be thinking that all of this sounds very idealistic, or out of touch with real people's lives, but many real people have decided to make huge changes in their lives. These changes may have been as a result of an internal shift or brought about by external circumstances like Brexit, or COVID, or death of a loved one. Changes that meant deferring gratification, challenging addictive or abusive patterns, or stepping out of cosy, established dynamics, places that reinforced their victimhood, places that gave a sense of the hopelessness of life. Nature can be a consciously focused catalyst for change in life. Nature provides the perfect non-judgemental mirror to inspire and question us. We are offered not only hope but symbols of survival and redemption, challenge and self-assurance, mastery and grace, along with metaphors for struggle and success, expressions of freedom and expansion.

The collective practices of *shinrin-yoku*, including the immersive experience of being in the woods, the exploration with the senses, and the invitation to slow everything down and simply breathe, all contribute not just towards physiological or psychological changes, but when fully engaged with, they can lead to profound insight and self-inventory. This *liminal state* establishes a new way of knowing and understanding the self, opening our eyes to choices that are pro-health and pro-emancipation. Regular sessions reinforce this new paradigm, and it is suggested that clients commit to a minimum of six sessions; although strong results may be achieved in a single session, it is important to back this up with additional input where possible and support the integration of learning and change.

Self-determination theory[123] and recent empirical research suggests that people who focus on extrinsic goals or aspirations, like wealth, power, status, fame, personal attractiveness, and social recognition, score lower on wellbeing markers, whereas those who focus on intrinsic values that are congruent with personal growth, such as self-acceptance, affiliation, community engagement, and physical health, record higher scores. Intrinsic life goals are more closely aligned with a person's psychological needs, which in turn are related to our basic survival needs.

Foundational to the establishment of the first Ecotherapy Project with Plymouth NHS in 2008, was a desire to create a tribal feel to the group based around Maslow's hierarchy of needs.[124] The focus was on participants trusting the group to meet their survival needs, not as individuals but as a bonding collective. We met one day a week for a whole year, and the participants were responsible for the construction of their shelter and gathering wood to make fire for warmth and hot water.

These very simple basic tasks were sufficient to elicit the therapeutic benefits of being in an outdoor setting, creating a new community where individuals felt recognised and acknowledged for their roles and their contributions, which were instantly tangible. Good communication was recognised as key to the success of these practical tasks. If you didn't get the shelter right, you would all get wet; if the fire wasn't tended, there would be no hot drinks or warmth. Contrast this with NHS interventions which were largely focused on drug administration, and non-demanding activities such as going shopping, playing pool, and trips to the cinema. These passive activities did not demand engagement from the clients and they switched off from life.

> I can vividly recall one day in January when we had been asked to cut down some second-growth conifers that had sprung up on Dartmoor. We were in a place called Dendle's Waste, a high, exposed, bleak expanse of featureless moorland which was being battered by a snow blizzard. Some members of the group were trying to get a fire going, but it was so cold that nothing would light, and so we all just sat there eating our lunch in the snowstorm, laughing at the absurdity of what we were doing – a memorable day!

Maslow's hierarchy is now 80 years old, and it felt important to add a higher frequency, or more refined model based on contemporary developments at the interface between positive psychology, anthropology, and evolutionary biology. The Human Givens model sits perfectly above Maslow's original theory and serves as a practical and empirical refinement for the contemporary therapeutic tribe structure within the Ecotherapy Project. This positive psychology model incorporates both self-protection and esteem motives from evolutionary biology and posits that if we meet the basic biological needs of the organism, i.e., treat humans as if they were animals and provide the most optimum habitat for that animal, then they will thrive, and not be subject to depression (my interpretation).

Originated by therapists Joe Griffin and Ivan Tyrell,[125] the Human Givens approach suggests that Nature has endowed us with universal emotional needs, and the best communities are the ones that satisfy these biological needs to ensure happiness, optimum functioning, and wellbeing. Nature has endowed us with a set of inner resources to meet those emotional needs, which include the capacity to dream, to build rapport (social engagement systems), and to have a long-term memory. I am a very big supporter of this approach as it acknowledges our intrinsic animal nature and has a universal appeal, not an exclusively Western-oriented perspective. It emphasises the important contribution that being in Nature can make to our overall well-being, particularly our mental health.

So to recap on health: we need to attend to our own unique relationship and intimacy with Nature as therapists and walk leaders, to ensure that we can provide the holding and therapeutic containment for our participants. We need some understanding of the flora and fauna of our patch; we need to have all of our risk assessments in place, and also understand the aims and intentions of the session(s), build reciprocity into our practice, remain flexible, spontaneous, intuitive, and open-minded about where this journey may take us, and never underestimate the healing powers of Nature.

Wild Apple Tree

Have you ever seen or encountered a wild apple tree? Apple trees are members of the rose family and have five petals to the flowers and five carpels or seed pods within the apple (cut one horizontally to see the beautiful five seed shape). There are two types of apple tree in the British countryside: the wild crab apple and the cultivated apple.

The native common wild crab apple, *Malus sylvestris*, has a profusion of small hard fruits in colours ranging from yellow through to green and red and combinations in between. Crab apples are also the only native apple tree of North America.

The overall shape of the tree is tall, round, and pleasing to the eye. It grows to about 30–40ft high. These trees stand strong, and the fruits make an excellent jelly or cordial with the addition of sufficient sugar to balance their tart flavour. It is always a joy to come across one of these ancient trees within the countryside, and to stop and spend time with it.

I like to watch the arrangements and patterns of its branches, and the procession of pinky-white buds and flowers that precede the formation of the fruits which grow in size throughout the summer, until in autumn the fruits fall and lie in profusion under the canopy. Once the leaves are shed, in winter we can see the very pleasing silhouette of the tree shape and formation. I encourage you to seek out these trees within your landscapes and spend some time with them, just looking and sensing, and enjoying.

The cultivated apple tree is also a strange and exciting pleasure to come across on our walks. These domestic apple trees have various etiological roots (excuse the pun!) and provenance. Some of them tend to be old residual trees left over from when the area was an orchard, and may well be varieties of ancient cider trees. Others may have grown from a seed dropped by a bird, or as I have witnessed alongside the main carriageway near me, a wide variety of beautiful apple trees of varying shapes, sizes, and colours which have undoubtedly grown from apple cores tossed out of car windows. It gives me so much pleasure to drive past these trees and see how they have adapted and found a niche in the no-man's-land beside the road.

If we get the opportunity to study these deviant escapees, we find their branches and stems so much thicker and stouter than the wild crab trees with their more slender branches. These cultivars look sturdy and their branch shape is unmistakeable. I have spent a considerable amount of my life climbing apple trees, hired by neighbours to pick their apples as a child, then pruning apple trees and working on the harvest of apples both here in the UK and in France. Orchards still excite me, the promise of rich lush fruits – Cox are my favourite.

Another thing worth noting is how the escapee trees start to revert back towards their feral ancestry; without the vigour of the rootstock, it is almost as if they have found their way back to the Mother Earth and can now be themselves – a powerful metaphor.

Forest bathing is an opportunity to recalibrate our sensory apparatus towards deeper love and appreciation of all beings, and slowing down to experience the personalities and details of trees and plants is such a rich and accessible rewarding activity, which leads us into a soul awakening that's impossible to describe but feels not only artistic, reverent, dreamy, uplifting, thought-provoking, sensual and happy, but also troubled.

I give the example of the apple tree, but it could have been thousands of other such phenomena that brings us to life. Try looking for lady's mantle *Alchemilla mollis* growing wild in the landscape and take a magnifying glass with you, and lose yourself for an hour just observing this exquisite jewel.

CHAPTER 8

Into the Forest

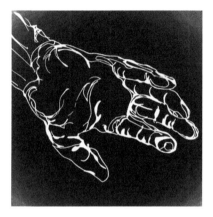

Before we get going, it's very important to state that I recommend people undertake a proper in-person training course before advertising themselves as forest bathing walk leaders. To repeat the message from the Introduction, this book is not a substitute for that essential training course; it is a companion to the training, exploring some of the themes in greater detail, and delving into some areas that form part of the larger picture.

How to choose a forest

Well, actually it's better to let the forest choose us, in an ideal world. However, sometimes practicalities need to be considered, so let's have a look at these and some of the criteria for a great venue for forest bathing. Although there are no hard and fast rules on this, it comes down to a variety of factors, and whilst there are no perfect forests, it's also true that we can do some forest bathing anywhere we find Nature, however small. Noise can be a distracting factor, but in some locations unavoidable, and so we find ways to zone out the sound, build it in, or just tune in to other sounds in Nature.

Do you have an existing area of forest that you know well? Is it the closest or most convenient one? Or is it an area of forest that you feel particularly drawn to each time you go for a walk? If it feels like a very special place to you, just check in whether you want to share that place with others or not. It took me a whole year of thinking and feeling and resting before I could decide on suitable venues for this work. There are quite a few amazing forests around me, but only two just felt right, like a good fit in so many ways – not just the convenience of parking, but more to do with the energy of the woods – the atmosphere felt friendly and welcoming and diverse.

Criteria will be different depending on the size and needs of the group, and, especially if you are working in a one-to-one session with a client, some of these rules do not apply (but others might – developing forest bathing experiences for a one-to-one session takes a very different trajectory). Some factors to consider are:

- size, aspect, function and terrain

- composition and biodiversity

- facilities and access

- any legal issues

- amount of footfall

- noise: traffic, planes, power lines, other users

- suitable routes matched to timescales

- purpose of session matching the energy of the woods.

Size, aspect, function, and terrain

Consider the size and shape of the forest. It's no good going round an area of woodland in ten minutes when it's a two-hour session, or setting off on a long trail that takes you miles away from the starting point and then having to retrace your steps (a circular walk is sometimes best but not always).

The aspect is the direction in which the forest faces. Quite often, the forest only exists because the land was deemed bad for agriculture, which might mean that it faces north and gets hammered by a bitter wind all day and is in the shadows from midday onwards.

What is the function of these woods? Are they primarily for commercial or for amenity use? If it's commercial, you might come along one day to find that the whole lot has been clear-felled – it happens quite frequently. If it's designated for amenity use, check that you won't be bombarded by joggers and cyclists, and whether you need to get permission for an event (see 'Legal issues' below).

The terrain must be suitable not only for walking but for sitting, standing, lying down, and perhaps for sitting in a circle. The terrain must be stable and safe. I did some training up in the Lake District and when I had looked at the woods on Google Earth, they just looked like lovely green fluffy balls, but when I went there for a recce the day before the course, the slope was very steep, and it was raining, and I was sliding down the path backwards – not ideal! Check the terrain is not too rocky, or boggy, or whether it has lots of steps and slopes. Has there been felling there recently so that lots of branches are all tangled up and impassable? How are the paths after rain? In another woodland that I worked in, the paths were great until it started raining, and then the clay turned the whole thing into a skating rink and I had to grab on to the trees to stay upright.

Composition

I could almost write a whole book on this one topic. Look for woods with some diversity, some mixtures of trees; it doesn't matter what they are, either conifer or broad leaf, just not monocrop (even non-stop oaks can be too much after a while). Shrubs and understorey trees are fabulous. In several of my local woods, there are crab apples and cherries, and they bring a crisp, fruity note to the woodland mix.

Also, a healthy woodland is a good place to start. Try to sense how the forest feels. It might have all the right components but not in the right proportions, or something is not quite gelling. It comes down to your intuitive sense and not a checklist of species. Biodiversity happens when woods find their optimum operating ambience, when the land remains undisturbed and the full plethora of wild species can grow harmoniously. Ancient woods have indicator species such as bluebells (*Hyacinthoides non-scripta*) that show that the ground and trees have remained undisturbed (for a minimum of 100 years preferably).

Facilities and access

Facilities can cover car parking, trails for wheelchair or mobility scooter use, toilets, a cafe, or shelter. Generally, we don't need much beyond a meeting point, usually a car park, and I tend to avoid busy or commercial venues, favouring woods with few or no facilities. Part of the process of rewilding *Homo sapiens* starts with eliminating some unnecessary comforts, distractions and conveniences. Of course, we always make exceptions depending on the needs of individuals within the group, but generally we keep it simple.

Access also needs to be considered. How will people get there? Is there a clear meeting point, adequate parking, or signposting to the start? If people can get lost, they absolutely will – despite all of your efforts, they will get lost and disappear, trust me.

Legal issues

These include insurances, permissions, and any boundary issues, restrictions, and other red tape that you may come across. Check the woods are open to the public (unless you have the very good fortune to have come to a private agreement with a landowner who is sympathetic to what you are offering – they do exist).

Permissions are a real problem these days. Agencies tend not to understand what we are doing, and can be overly cautious or too greedy, or bombard us with too much admin – it's ridiculous. There needs to be an easier decision-making process for establishing the value and benefits of forest bathing on site for landowners, and a greater degree of professionalism and standards so that we are not at the mercy of various policies that are not Nature focused, but fear or money focused.

Footfall

This is important for two main reasons. First, if there are loads of people walking by, some participants may feel a bit inhibited to really explore the relationship with Nature and the vulnerability of it. Second, I find large numbers of visitors have a significant impact on the forest energy. Big wide paths squash and compress tree roots and compact the soil; there can be litter, or within the first hundred feet of the entrance lots of dog poo, sadly. (We do try to pick up the litter if we can.)

I was once instructing a group of teachers in a very busy area, with a massive car park, visitor centre, and wide overused trails with huge life-size Gruffalo sculptures. It was so busy that I needed to escape, so the next day I agreed to meet the group about a mile further along the large forest, in an area with a forest worker's cottage and some mature trees and lawns set within a lush forested valley. There was nobody there, we had the place to ourselves the whole day, and the group realised that they had never been there before, although just up the road, because they assumed the need to be near the toilets. They unanimously agreed to look into hiring a portaloo for the days they were out with children, and coming up to that part of the forest in future, as it was so quiet, still, and cool, and remained mysterious.

Noise, traffic and planes, and other potential intrusions

These things are part and parcel of our lives, so we cannot avoid them, particularly if our woods border a busy road or a flat area without hills to muffle traffic noise. I once found some ideal woods in the New Forest well away from the many large, noisy roads, only to discover it was under the flightpath of the airport, but nobody else seemed to notice as we sat under the old oaks.

Matching routes to timescales and to participants

I know this seems obvious, but it is an important factor to consider in the way that you choreograph your routes. How long will this walk around the woods take with a group? How often will you stop to take breaks and do exercises, talk, look at things, get lost, and maybe have a change of route completely?

Most of these things get smoothed out over time; the more time you spend in the woods, the more accurately you can predict timings, and make readjustments and allow for contingencies. Have a selection of suitable routes for different groups, and be comfortable with changing your route at any moment. Remember it takes far longer to walk round with a group than an individual, so don't rush things or be over ambitious, but allow for a range of locations and focal points within the forest.

Energy matching

The final point is quite important: matching the energy and needs of your group with the energy and needs of the forest. What is the purpose of this session? How do you want it to play out so that people benefit from this experience? It is also important to consider the needs of the forest, and whether you feel welcomed there and held by the trees. Establishing the purpose of the session may inform your choice of walk or which forest to visit. If we know what the client group is expecting, then we can start to dream the walk alive, and this process will take on a life of its own. However, we can only do this when we have a good, thorough knowledge and intimate relationship with the forest we are intending to visit.

We also need to carefully consider the follow-up. What happens after that session? How does the meeting with the forest impact on participants' lives and how can we support that thread of connection? So much of our lives are only about superficial gratifying experiences that intersperse the quiet desperation and struggle of life, so perhaps we have a responsibility to offer people ways to maintain this connection and grow it. Perhaps we need to check in with them post-walk, to help cultivate habits of visiting Nature and develop the practice of reverence and joy. If we can help people grow this connection into a lifelong, heartfelt relationship, then we have done a good deed. Spending time in Nature does not equate to connecting to Nature – attitude, conscious connection, and intention are key to this new paradigm, a willingness to explore our spiritual roots in the woods, in beauty and vitality.

Ecological knowledge

I am definitely a bit old school on this point, but I feel with the growing trend of therapy outdoors that practitioners would benefit from having a working knowledge of the plant and animal communities they are accessing and passing through. If you have a counselling, psychotherapy, or psychology degree, you may feel adequately trained to lead clients out into the woods, but would you want a botanist or forest worker to be your therapist? I do believe that we need to develop skills in both disciplines to be at our most effective, for the following two reasons.

Metaphorical/spiritual insights

When we have even a basic knowledge of the key tree and plant species in our woods, then we have a richer and more comprehensive depth to our work, which adds another dimension to the therapeutic narratives that we work with. Not all forest bathing practitioners have a counselling or therapy qualification, and I stress that these are not essential in order to lead forest bathing walks, as we understand that the forest and Nature do the healing. However, if we know the names and habits of some plants, and we know a little bit about that beetle that crossed the path, we enrich the experience so much. I suggest that new practitioners learn three new plants or animals every year.

When we begin to see how all the various organisms and networks fit together, we feel an even deeper sense of awe for the forest and its inhabitants. We are fascinated by the mycelial networks below the soil, and the huge variety of fruiting bodies that spring up above the soil, on the trees and dead wood. We love the magical world of the mini-beasts and the elusive lichens, and we gaze up through that shimmering green canopy with gratitude.

When we get to know just a few of the forest denizens, we begin to have a curiosity that grows to learn more and an understanding of how certain significant encounters with Nature may have a metaphorical or spiritual significance. 'Spiritual' feels like a personal message in Nature language, a kind of portent or symbol that carries specific weight or significance at a given moment, or related to the intention that we arrived with. Not everything we see has this, don't get too carried away; it's more of a heightened super-reality feeling.

Similarly, we can sense a Nature-mirroring example that connects closely to our ongoing dialogue with the client's issues or concerns, whether these have been explicitly stated or left unsaid. Sometimes our intuition is drawn towards something without knowing why, and we can simply notice something and point it out, leaving it up to the client to decipher, react, or comment on it. We don't lead that conversation, except where we notice a direct correlation with the immediate topic in conversation, where we want to tentatively draw comparisons with Nature, or make observations of an example from Nature that bolsters an idea or theory. Metaphors abound in Nature, and we can dilute the narrative by applying them too often, but at just the appropriate moment they can lead to insight and be very catalytic in terms of personal growth and reframing perspectives.

When we are offered these metaphors, they can speak to us so directly that either we feel empowered or we decide that we are not ready for change and choose to suppress the image and its message that we have received at a subconscious and conscious level, particularly if it relates to death, the harbinger of change and transformation (see the Death card from the tarot deck and its symbolism).

Honouring and respecting Nature as if it mattered
It can feel abstract and mawkish to consciously pay attention to Nature. Most of us are isolated from any sense of direct dependence on Nature, and therefore have no imperative to make more than a token effort to care for the planet, until we are faced with imminent oblivion.

If we can start now to cultivate Nature-revering practices, as New Age or sentimental as that might seem, we can embed habits that have a direct impact on our current zeitgeist of responsibility-free consumption. Things are changing, and change is driven from the bottom upwards, although perceived as from the top downwards. It is the consumer who dictates the politics of consumption, demanding that companies become more green, more accountable for human rights issues, that they use less plastic packaging etc., with government eventually following with new legislation. Patagonia are an example of an inspiring visionary organisation, who have set aside their profits to be returned back to Nature projects, have adopted many environmentally friendly policies, and are currently supporting a major campaign to protect one of Europe's last wild rivers in Albania.

On an individual scale, by learning more about the plants and animals all around us and by befriending them, we are showing a commitment to respecting and engaging with our ecosystems. If we wander around oblivious to these individual species, their unique characteristics, and their unique medicine, we are in danger of becoming a part of the old exploitative narrative, simply using Nature without caring for it, or even knowing anything about it.

Each plant, each tree, each mushroom, and each animal has a very important lesson or medicine for us. This is why species extinction is such a huge issue, because we begin to lose not only their wisdom and gifts but also the fabric of the web; the interconnecting nodes disappear and the whole collapses. Learning about each member of our community, their names, habits, preferences, how they thrive, what they feed on, makes a massive difference to us and to them. Again it comes back to sacred relationship, honouring our kinship and family of all beings.

Choosing a forest

Hopefully, you can find a forest that is happy to teach you and to host you. It's great to spend as much time there as you can, so go there in the morning, the afternoon (particularly at dusk and dawn, the two magic in-between times), visit in the night, in the rain, the snow, the heat of the day, and in all the moods that you experience within yourself. Gradually, you will develop such a good bond with the woods, and yet always be surprised by some new vista, or visitor.

Once you feel really familiar with your woods and have perhaps found some special places that you like to hang out, you may get a sense of where you would like to visit with others, and so a route or plan is loosely formed. Ask permission from the forest and seek to get the trees on your side – after all, they are doing the work; we are just the guides and witnesses, and occasionally translators. It's important not to become rigid or fixed on routes; ideally, they would change every day as the woods are different every day. Please allow for complete spontaneity – what's the worst thing that could happen?

Forest bathing forests have lots of sensory exchange, lots of awe moments, lots of holding, some good stories, some grand-mother trees, and if we are very lucky, a stream running through them. Coming out in all weathers and seeing what's going on is no different from meeting up with a good friend for a chat, and a chance to talk about what is going on in life together. All forests have value and something to offer us; even the densely packed conifer plantation has something to teach us, some love to share. Please don't be judgemental and choosy over areas of woods, but keep an open mind to the possibilities of each location. It may be just what a client needs.

All woodlands are unique all over the world, even in the same county with the same soils, the exact composition and configuration of the individual species and the atmosphere will vary considerably. This can be to our advantage in determining which woods to visit on a particular day with a particular client or group.

When I am doing my ecotherapy work, I wait for an image of an area to pop into my mind whilst I'm having a shower, driving, cooking, or washing up. I then go and sit with that place and see if it feels right, wait there in silence until I get a positive energy from that place. Then I meet there with the client and just watch what happens without any sense of a plan. I might intuitively take something with me on the day, like kit for making a fire, or a blanket, or my hand lens; it varies.

It may be useful to think of the different areas or different little places within the landscape as acupuncture needles. In Chinese medicine, illness can occur when our energy channels (meridians) get blocked, or where heat builds up in an organ connected to these internal pathways. Inserting acupuncture needles at key points on the body helps to release or restimulate blocked or stagnant energy. We can apply the same principle within the landscape, with each specific place acting upon a specific aspect of the person's being; a dark, foreboding, or cold place might be just what they need to trigger a shift either psychically, physiologically, psychologically or emotionally.

Even specific plants can be somehow more energetic, more available, as each plant and animal has a signature tune, a kind of magnetic field of resonance. When we come close to these phenomena, we can sense their individual frequencies, and their close presence can serve to rebalance or retune our own internal microclimates and help to restore us back towards homeostasis. This is simply a more direct way of imbibing the essence of the plant or animal and allowing its medicine to work with us. This is part of the notion of active benignity, that there is movement towards us when we need it, when we are ready to receive it.

If this all sounds a bit far-fetched, unscientific, or 'woo woo', I think it's because of how we have mostly lost our refined attunement to these states and connections. I say mostly, because if you were to ask a range of ordinary people, you will find that many of them have reported an encounter with Nature that took them to a different feeling state beyond that which they were suffering. Nature cannot contradict the laws of the Universe, one of which is our right to free will and determinism; however, occasionally there is a need for stronger interventions to assist us on another plane.

Active benignity

Is Nature inherently aggressive towards us? That doesn't mean parents protecting their young or animals trying to eat you – it's not personal. The answer would seem to be no, not inherently aggressive. Is Nature simply neutral, then? Just getting on with its own business, like us? I think there's a bit of that going on; Nature is largely opportunistic, and so evolution and survival stuff is happening whether we are around or not. So yes, a bit neutral.

Is Nature inherently friendly and positive? I like to think that yes, in many ways it is. I like to indulge the idea that if and when things are aligned, Nature actually wants to support us in some way. There is an unconditional love that is exuded by Nature, and that is the message that I get when I am out there and open to receiving it. Plants and animals have strong life forces all oscillating at different frequencies, and because we have within us the memories of these evolutionary stages, we are affected by their presence.

For example, the poisonous plants have such a strong energetic presence that it is worth getting as close to one as you are permitted, and to simply sit in silence for a while. They have a large, old aura of quiet power, and we can paradoxically heal from being in their presence. We don't imbibe them; we just sit still with them. The so-called entheogens are poisonous plants that have been known for many generations to have divinatory and visionary powers, and some toxic effects too. Psychedelics are powerful allies, but ordinary plants like nettle and monkshood have incredible properties. Nettle you can ingest, but monkshood you must *never* ingest – it will kill you, or make you extremely ill; just meditate with it near you, observe all its beauty and magnificence. Feel its energetic signature. It is a powerful homeopathic remedy for fear of death.

If we can trust Nature to be benign and benevolent, we develop such a different perception of even our gardens and parks; we simply need to ask for help, and offer a little gift back if we feel inclined to. It is unconditional love that is shared; no matter how abusive we are to her, Nature comes back with abundance and grace.

Choreographing a route

As I mentioned, if possible, allow the route of your walk to simply suggest itself, and always be open to it changing at a moment's notice. If you become too certain of the route, you risk missing out on any spontaneous happenings on the day. If you were to be completely spontaneous, then you may risk not knowing what's going to happen for the whole walk and perhaps miss a few things. That may be fine too, but it isn't an excuse for just turning up completely unprepared without having previously checked out the site before, and winging it.

Some structure allows you to relax, knowing that there are places that will hold the group, and what happens in between is open to the day, such as visiting a hawthorn that's in bloom to smell its blossoms, or having a break by a stream that catches the light around midday.

A final word: don't try to fit too much in; periods of walking in silence are probably the most beneficial thing we can do. Trust, trust, trust, and let go.

CHAPTER 9

Thresholds

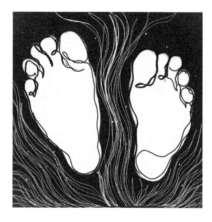

A threshold or portal is a point of transition between one world and another. Crossing it is more than simply entering a place of transformation, it somehow marks a point of no return, an embodied stepping over, stepping through, or falling, so it can be both voluntary or involuntary (which may also be subconsciously voluntary). It can be a consciously chosen or recognised physical expression of a gateway within the landscape, or more of a mythical change of pressure. Crossing a threshold is often marked by a shift away from the material world, the world of thoughts and preoccupation with the modalities of everyday existence, and a descent into the world of pure experience, of instincts and unarticulated feelings. We experience the unlimited potential of Nature, unmediated by thinking or labelling, uncensored in the same ways that our dreams are, giving rise to uninhibited expressions of *psyche* and *eros*.

Thresholds are often physical gateways into the woods, or the start of a footpath. They can take the form of stiles, gates, gaps in a wall, a bridge over a stream, a panel missing from a fence, where the wire was cut, or a specific change in terrain or vegetation. Quite often, a threshold is found created by trees and bushes; an overhanging branch creates an arched opening into the

135

woods. In one of my special places, the threshold involves walking along a low wall between a stream and a bog, then stepping between a cleft tree to enter the magic kingdom. In the city once, I was driving around and I stopped near a high fence. I found a gap in the fence and squeezed through, immediately finding myself amongst fecundity and abundance, the proliferation of seeds and flowers and wildness reclaiming a derelict site. Suddenly, I was in another world, as if I had gone through a gateway from children's stories, or stepped through the wardrobe.

Choosing a cleft tree is an invaluable symbolic passage point for entry to other realms, and one that reminds me of the story of the goddess Inanna and her sister, Ereshkigal, goddess of the underworld. In the Sumerian version of the myth, Inanna decides to pay her sister a visit in the underworld and hammers at the gates to be let through. Neti the gatekeeper reports this to Ereshkigal who instructs him to let her through, but to narrow the entrances at the seven gates to the underworld. At each gate, Inanna is forced to strip away more and more of her royal garments and jewellery until eventually, when she arrives before her sister, she is naked and unadorned.

In this myth, Inanna has been interpreted as representative of the ego and the arrogance of our entitlement to wealth and power, which is inevitably stripped from us all at death. At each narrowing of the gates, corresponding to our cleft in the tree, we are forced to shed another layer of our armour and ego defence until we are reduced down to our bare selves. So, as we enter the realms of Nature, of Sylvanus, we are reminded to be humble and leave some extraneous baggage behind.

Types of threshold

It is possible to dedicate your own threshold point if one does not present itself. Maybe choose two closely growing trees and pass between them, or go under a branch, or jump across a stream. Find your own unique transition point for the area that you inhabit. Sometimes, particularly at night, the mere act of stepping outside our door constitutes a threshold, from the artificial environment of the house to the wildness of the dark.

An event or encounter with Nature can also often serve as a threshold, a way of shifting our awareness to the other/outer realms, especially if it's sudden and unexpected. Sometimes we may need to traverse multiple thresholds in one session, and this can give us a sense of lightness and elation, of shedding skins as we step beyond our limitations. The Irish poet, author, and philosopher John O'Donohue wrote so beautifully about this threshold experience, likening it to an awakening, with the arrival of spring catching us out in our long-held winter mentality, leaving us vulnerable as we 'negotiate the challenge of the threshold'.[126]

> The etymology of 'threshold' is interesting, and its true meaning is obscure and lost in time, but it derives from Greek, Latin, and Sanskrit words meaning to rub, thresh, grind, or wear away. The time of threshing the harvested grain was an extremely important festival in the pagan/agrarian calendar, a time for people to come together to celebrate, as they still do in some parts of the world like the Czech Republic and Italy.
>
> Raw grain is brought into the threshing room, crossing the threshold from the plant domain, and emerges from the rotating quernstone transformed into flour that can be cooked and eaten. In this way, this rubbing away is important in our lives as a necessary renewal process and in the removal of our hardened outer husks.

O'Donohue further suggests that when these thresholds appear, they are a challenge that requires 'courage and a sense of trust in whatever is emerging'.[125] This is where the grounding of the therapist is critical. We may no longer find ourselves standing on the solid ground of our familiar and well-worn life, and are now stepping out into the unknown, just like the image of the Fool from the tarot deck stepping off the cliff. As forest bathing leaders and practitioners, it is important that we can witness and support this metamorphic process.

It is often easy to assume that these simple gestures of crossing thresholds in the woods are purely symbolic, but they can have deep, psychological import for the subconscious processes that resonate with Nature. These journeys or crossings can be unsettling and can initiate a process of reflection or self-interrogation, and become a catalyst for learning and change, which 'often involves messy journeys back, forth and across conceptual terrain'.[127]

Thresholds can be real physical features marking the entrance (the 'en-trance') of the forest. They can also be found within the forest, and we may seek out multiple such thresholds on occasion to signify some cleansing process. We may choose to acknowledge them with our participants overtly, or we may simply internally recognise the stepping over into the other world, without the need to bring it up.

One exercise which proves popular with students is to ask each participant to find a natural object and to place all their worries and woes in the natural object and then leave it behind before stepping over the threshold. They are invited, of course, to pick it up again when they return if they need it, or throw to it into the stream as we cross a bridge entering the woods, for example.

Another small conscious ritual is to ask someone to be the voice of the forest and to stand by the threshold. If this is a gate, it is kept closed, then when each person approaches, it is opened and they are welcomed through the entrance. This ritual may be repeated on leaving the woods, and may be accompanied by a small gift of words or a natural object like an acorn, chestnut, or stick.

This exercise was combined to dramatic effect one day with the cleft tree threshold. A student who was a Druid had brought with him a beautiful handmade pouch of dried flowers from his garden, and he stood by the cleft tree and invited us across slowly, in silence, each of us picking a flower from the pouch as we squeezed through the gap. The effect had me in tears; it was exquisite and set the tone for the rest of the magical day.

Liminality

A concept closely linked with thresholds is liminality, meaning 'relating to a transitional or initial stage of a process' or 'occupying a position at, or on both sides of, a boundary or threshold'.[128] It has been suggested that crossing over the threshold into the forest is a process of liminality, of going between the worlds and discovering hidden truths.

Liminality and liminal space are terms borrowed from anthropology, specifically the work of ethnographer and folklorist Arnold van Gennep. His book *The Rites of Passage* was published in 1909, wherein he coined the term *liminal* to describe the three distinct stages of a rites of passage experience, claiming that 'such rituals marking, helping, or celebrating individual or collective passages through the cycle of life or of nature exist in every culture, and share a specific three-fold sequential structure'.[129]

- A pre-liminal state (or rites of separation): This stage involves a metaphorical 'death', as the initiate is forced to leave something behind by breaking with previous practices and routines, and lifestyles (as in the stripping back process I alluded to earlier).

- Liminal rites (or transition rites): Two characteristics are considered essential to these rites. First, the rite 'must follow a strictly prescribed sequence, where everybody knows what to do and how'. Second, everything must be done 'under the authority of a master of ceremonies'. The destructive nature of this rite allows for considerable changes to be made to the identity of the initiate. This middle stage (when the transition takes place) becomes an actual passing through the threshold that marks the boundary between two phases, two worlds, and into as yet unknown realms.

The term liminality was used to describe this passage. It is characterised by the initiate being isolated from the rest of society, and stripped of their identity, gender, and often their clothes too. This middle, in-between stage, is regarded as:

> a suspended state of partial understanding, or 'stuck place', in which understanding approximates to a kind of 'mimicry' or lack of authenticity. Insights gained by learners as they cross thresholds can be exhilarating but might also be unsettling, requiring an uncomfortable shift in identity, or, paradoxically, a sense of loss.[130]

- Post-liminal rites (or rites of incorporation): During this stage, the initiate is gradually reincorporated into society with a new identity, as a 'new' being.[131]

The anthropologist Victor Turner later confirmed the liminality structure of van Gennep's work through his fieldwork living with the Ndembu tribe in Zambia; he observed numerous rites of passage and wrote about them in his excellent book *The Forest of Symbols*.[132] Turner argued that what was relevant for the Ndembu had a far-reaching significance across society in general, and his work sought to form these links between Ndembu rites of passage and broader cultural experience.

Turner recognised the importance of these in-between periods, human responses to liminal experience, and the way that liminality influences personality: 'the sudden foregrounding of agency, and the sometimes dramatic tying together of thought and experience'.[133] Liminal stages are marked by a sense of ambiguity and disorientation, and anchoring exercises within the forest may serve to help 'ground' a person or group within their somatic experience, as they make this transitional journey but have not yet arrived at their new status.

The post-liminal or integrative stage can lead towards a sense of transformation and a new narrative about life. Forest therapy supports this ontological enquiry process through the immersive and sensorial experiences that provide a biophilic container for the dissolution of the former self and redundant aspects of the psyche that need recycling. This corresponds to Carl Jung's idea of a *temenos* or sanctuary to protect the vulnerability of the individuation process. The forest furnishes us with historical and subliminal sanctuary as well as offering us the optimum physical and metaphorical model for dynamic systems-related change.

Finally, Turner indicates that these liminal states cannot be maintained indefinitely, and at some point, these liminal communities (or 'communitas' as Turner calls them) must dissolve and return to the surrounding social structure. Communitas consist of individuals who collectively experience the camaraderie of rites of passage experiences.[134] Integration of post-liminal experiences can take time, and it is useful to have simple nature-based rituals to serve as mediators and reminders of the diminishing intensity of the initial ontological shift.

The traversing of thresholds can be a precarious and unsettling shift into the turbulent and unknown waters beneath the surface of consciousness, and into the existential or soul enquiry into life and purpose, and being and acceptance. As John O'Donohue reminds us:

> To sense and trust this primeval acceptance can open a vast spring of trust within the heart. It can free us into a natural courage that casts out fear and opens up our lives to become voyages of discovery, creativity, and compassion. No threshold need be a threat, but rather an invitation and a promise.[135]

It becomes evident that having the capacity to offer several sessions can help with integration processes and build Nature connection practices that affirm and anchor the effects of liminal experiences. Small rituals can offer a powerful reminder of key insights and feelings of empowerment. Embedding nature rituals into everyday life serves to reinforce the changes and become a resource for further turbulent times.

Nature as Lover, Paramour

Our bodies were designed to be in love with Nature, in union, our senses primed for the electric quiver of connection and the blur of exquisite diaphanous ecstasy. Nature beckons to us over and over, a siren song, dancing naked before our eyes and pulling us back deeper into the primal embrace that we were born from.

How many times have you felt that seductive breeze on your skin, or the lap of water around your thighs, the radiant sun demanding your surrender and soft, lush strokes of wet vegetation on your bare legs and arms. I count myself lucky to have experienced such paroxysmal joys in my life, and yet recently I seem to be yearning for those sensual moments more than ever, to fall into my lover's arms, to cling to her, to surrender myself entirely to her, a willing servant and acolyte, and to say my prayers, cherish what I have received since birth, since my first steps, to gorge myself on her fruits, to smell the familiar intoxicating sweetness of the moist soil, that melliferous, yet putrefying bouquet of home.

Sensing how time is ever precious, no room for dithering, the need to be reminded of purpose (and of no purpose), of belonging, to be strongly here, be alive, and to fully feel all that life proffers and exult in that sweet place of love and desire for the earth and the blanket of leaves my lover has strewn before me. Making love with the Earth is a tender thing, and to do so we can accept the invitation to fully inhabit the body, the living flesh, the beckoning whispers; the songs and spells of the night's creatures demand that of us, 'embody me again they call', sending our consciousness to every nook and cranny of our physical form, out into the cool, dense, swirling enchantment of the night, enlivening our primal sensing appendages. We must come with humility and grace and humour, and risk being enveloped by something greater – that ecstasy that Rumi felt, the union with the one.

When the unsettled mind focuses on there being an event or thought and an observer, this then sometimes splits reality, objectivity asserts dominance, a duality then occurs which robs us of this raw visceral touching and tasting. We deserve to be fully embodied, to relegate the mind, because as Nan Shepherd discovers, 'no metaphor, transparent, or light as air, is adequate. The body is not made negligible, but paramount. Flesh is not annihilated but fulfilled. One is not bodiless, but essential body.'[136] Her semi-erotic prose describes how the Cairngorm mountains (surely the harshest environmental habitat of the British Isles) become this metaphorical and physical lover, and this intimate passionate relationship is described in a luxurious and sensual eulogy to Nature in its rawest and therefore most rewarding form.

So much of what is posted on social media about forest bathing either relates or depicts nice pictures of forests and sunsets, or lengthy reports about how good Nature is for us. I'm always left with a strong sense that much of that imagery and discussion neatly avoids what we consider to be Nature's base instincts for procreation and food. It's great to see projects that benefit Nature and spread good news about the rewilding efforts and conservation work that is so necessary. However, a conversation or narrative about Nature absolutely needs to include a reclaiming of our sexuality, which has been hijacked by advertising and media to sell us things that we don't need.

Our innocent ground of acceptance and love was replaced with shame long before all of this, and it seems that we have been left with such a legacy of distorted, contaminated, and deviant perspectives on love and sexuality that we can no longer even discuss it except on some late-night television documentaries. It's great to see so many people reclaiming their sexuality and their right to express themselves free of the fetters of conditioned cultural responses.

The sexual energy of Nature is the awakening of our inherent creativity which is a channel of inspiration and limitless energy latent within the Cosmos. Nature offers us another route to reawaken that latent energy or force, but we have to feel safe to invite it back in again. In forest bathing, we do not consciously evoke our sexuality through exercises, but practitioners should have an awareness of how these invitations to slow down, notice, and re-attune the senses will inevitably lead towards greater awareness of bodily driven sensations and feelings, and be prepared for possible strong emotional outcomes. Connecting deeply to Nature is an intimate experience, a sensual experience – let's embrace that.

Our primary sexual relationship with the land is a spiritual relationship, an earth-soul feeling of sublimation and ego dissolution, of merging with the sacred essence of all life, sharing our organic animal selves with the myriad creatures so that Nature becomes both the invitation and means for the release and being totally embodied and totally atomised, merged, temporarily in nirvana. I think that is a part of the attraction with open water swimming: the immersion into the fluid, under the big sky, and the ritual shedding of lots of suffocating clothes gives us this release from mortality and elevates consciousness by this sublimation to the wild flowing juices of the land.

Maybe the next time you are in Nature and it feels appropriate, see if you can consciously notice whether you can attune your sexuality to the landscape – I trust you to find the best way to do that, but symbols are powerful, intention is powerful, and movement is powerful. Cast off those distorted images and values, and have a joyful and sensual play and see what happens. Love yourself and the wild parts will find their way to express this release. Water, light, sound, play, sensual slow exploration and delight, relaxing body parts gently, inviting a mingling and flow – maybe it's a great big hearty oak tree, or a dark yew tree, or a cave, or a waterfall, or just a feeling of being on the earth, lying in a park. Smell and our primitive sensory touch mechanisms really love this awakening, but it can't be forced. Making love with the Earth can also come to us in our dreams.

On our Nature forums, let's start having more conversations about not just our sexuality but also about many other taboo topics like love, death, decay, and defecation, and let's not forget the taboo of discussing mental health in Nature.

CHAPTER 10

A Polyphony of The Senses

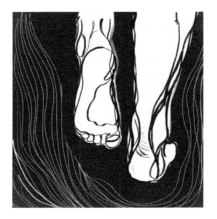

The whole skin has this delightful sensitivity; it feels the sun, it feels the wind running inside one's garment, it feels water closing on it as one slips under – the catch in the breath, like a wave held back, the glow that releases one's entire cosmos, running to the ends of the body as the spent wave runs out upon the sand. This plunge into the cold water of a mountain pool seems for a brief moment to disintegrate the very self; it is not to be borne: one is lost: stricken: annihilated. Then life pours back.

NAN SHEPHERD[137]

Life is a sensuous journey; our memories are built upon our sensual experiences of the world, experiences which are novel, yet investigated through psyche and the accumulated ancient perceptual knowledge that honed our senses as sharp calibrated tools. *Shinrin-yoku* is deliberately focused on awakening and engaging the senses fully in the forest environment, and exploring how our senses respond to all the myriad exotic and sensuous stimuli of our natural surroundings.

By enlivening and engaging the senses fully, we feel more alive, we physically expand; it's like somehow our auras expand out towards the horizon, we become more present in the moment and more connected to something bigger than us which feels calming, soothing, and uplifting too. Our mood is shifted into the positive when the senses are being stimulated, whether it's vision, touch, sound, smell, or taste.

There are numerous caveats to this statement, and we must primarily be attuned to the needs and limits of our clients in this. For some, opening up the senses can bring back trauma and pain, and be too overwhelming, and yet tentatively isolating and exploring one sense can also be a way to bypass the trauma and allow expansion and connection to arise in a healing way, without denying any reality.

A successful forest bathing session will illuminate, amplify, or electrify the senses, and recalibrate the sensitivity of each one. As therapists and practitioners, being in the woods is an opportunity to remember that when we are in direct contact with the other-than-human Nature, particularly the cocooning embrace of the forest, for all the faculties we have in order to 'make sense' of our environment, the forest has exactly the same senses to gauge, read, meet, and connect with us. The sentient arboreal matrix can see, hear, feel, touch, taste, and smell our presence. Its invisible tendrils reach out and delicately explore our succulent returning bodies.

Living in urban or semi-urban locations, and having employment that requires us to be in a certain place at a certain time and perform a specialist role whatever the profession, means the majority of us subconsciously suppress the full extent of our sensory awareness in order to slot into the daily rhythm of life, and filter out the onslaught of sensory stimuli that may overwhelm us if we remain too open. Commuting can also be a negative sensory over-stimulus.

It is extraordinary the lengths we have to go to, to suppress and straitjacket our unfettered emotions and sensations. Somehow in the corralling of our more socially disapproved emotions like anger, grief, and sadness, our higher spirits, our exuberant, wild, curious, infinite expressions of life, are also dragged down, and lie bound and gagged in the basement. When we come to the woods or beach, mountain, or desert, we can then let go and allow our senses to stretch out fully to the horizon, to find infinite vibrational textural expression. Nature is restorative partly due to the sensory permissiveness of its invitation.

Our senses are very much our wild primitive selves, and are so censored and under-utilised in ordinary consciousness. Our senses have been the key to us becoming successful hunter-gatherers, i.e., one that doesn't get eaten themselves. We have an extraordinary capacity to perceive beyond the boundaries of flesh, way out into the ether, we can detect what is near, and what is a threat or a source of food. We have the capacity to detect whether someone is staring at us from behind (more about this later). We can detect the presence of particles down to parts per billion – that's a single drop in a swimming pool.

In a 1995 University of Lausanne experiment that became known as 'The Sweaty T-shirt' experiment, Claus Wedekind's team was exploring the role of olfaction in detecting major histocompatability complex (MHC). A group of male students was asked to wear and sleep in the same T-shirts for two nights, and then those T-shirts were each placed in identical boxes and offered to a group of women to smell and indicate their preferences. The women chose the shirts of the men with the MHC that would balance out their own immune systems.[138]

Here is the key thing about the senses: they are both an integral part of our survival instincts and evolved predator skills, and they are also how our souls can experience materiality and corporality. So just as each sense in its own way is a gateway between our external perceived reality and our internal assimilation of data/stimuli, so too the senses are a portal between this world and other evolved realms of consciousness.

Our senses are the prism through which the soul seeks to understand the journey of incarnation. These senses are the portals of communication from stimuli to source and back. A reciprocal recognition of pure Spirit expressed through multitudinous creative forms. Each soul has a fascination with the sensory tangible version of life expression and the tentative and often fraught process of physical incarnation. It gives us a remarkable evolutionary insight to learn about how each sense works, how we perceive, and that intricate communion between what is perceived 'outside' of us and how we interpret that, the processing and decrypting of so much sensory information, and then how we measure, assess, and respond. Our sensory faculties are more closely aligned with our phylogenetic instincts, primitive and pure, and closer to Nature, rather than existing above it.

I want to distinguish that what I am referring to here is our *sensory* awareness, separate from our capacity to perceive, which is sensory input plus cultural influence plus memory plus brain chemistry. For example, advertisements seek to place an image or an idea in our mind without any conscious filtering. Pure sensory awareness exists before mental interpretation can categorise the experience, and it is the duty of the forest bathing walk leader to introduce exercises and phenomena that can elude this reductive perceptual bias, thus steering a participant towards an unprejudiced primary connection where the novel deployment of the senses suddenly opens up our true relationship with life. A simple example of this is the use of the 10x magnifying hand lens to gaze down on small mosses and liverworts.

Each of the senses is reliant on specialist cells that interact with the environment to convey information from the surface back to the corresponding parts of the brain for processing; the body then physiologically adjusts to that incoming data, independent of our conscious perceptual interpretations. We have our five outward-oriented senses of touch, taste, smell, sight, and hearing, and our bodies process internal somatosensory experiences based on billions of receptors located throughout the body,[139] giving us our vestibular, interoception, and proprioception senses that let us know who we are and where we are relative to our surroundings.

The senses are designed to work together synaesthetically, to create a three- or four-dimensional map of our surroundings and the subtle energies that impinge on that space. We live in a largely visually dominant world; image is all, and the media and marketing industries have been exploiting the visual appeal of products ever since Freud first identified our neuroses. (Of course, fashion has existed a lot longer than that, its purpose being to convey a visual message to attract or repel attention, signify status and the all-important 'sex appeal'.)

We are increasingly bombarded with cunningly deceptive images and accompanying slogans that try to persuade us we would have a much better life with product 'X' than without it. The visual image captures our attention so quickly that it bypasses sensory filters and tests. Visual imagery and auditory messaging have profound impacts at the undetected, subliminal level. Sight and sound can be engaged from a distance, unlike the other senses of touch, taste, and smell. We are susceptible to this visual and auditory assault since our primitive radar relies on these senses as our early warning system – perhaps that's why they are placed highest in the body. Advertisers fully comprehend both the mechanics of sight and perception and how the psychology of desire speaks to our post-arboreal duality homesickness blues.

This overloading with targeted imagery causes severe problems for the apparatus of perception, and the analysis and categorisation of meaning. The image of a car bursting out of an advertising hoarding is superficially abstract, then we overlay an understanding that it's a two-dimensional image, then we see the words 'Autumn sale', and we make an automatic assignation of meaning: this is a car, it denotes status, it's for sale, and now there's an offer on, so it's cheaper. All of that takes place in milliseconds at a subconscious level, without us needing to think.

One of the key roles in the evolutionary development of the brain is the detection of food (energy). It's no coincidence that the brain and the mouth are in proximity in most animals – in fact, the gut brain drove the development of the secondary head brain to control which nutrients were entering the mouth[140] (see Chapter 13, The Savage Self, for more details).

Visual overstimulation is now a serious addiction in modern societies, with an over-triggering of the brain's reward centres and dopamine release from viewing increasing levels of multi-consumption 'pornography'. But we are designed to be reading our environment in such a different way, and our Palaeolithic physiologies have not kept pace with our technological develop-ment and industrialised lifestyles, so that we suffer in a state of hyperarousal, our delicate sensory radars jammed with mass information overload.

Our primitive space-defining properties have been insidiously hijacked in order to keep us on board with the game. When we surrender ourselves to natural surroundings, we notice it doesn't take very long for that constant visual overstimulation and information processing frenzy to at last drop back down to a healthy pace and restful level of stimuli that enables us to function effectively at the biologically appropriate tasks we were designed to do. These are things like:

- looking for food and water

- avoiding becoming food

- bonding with the tribe

- seeking a mate and reproducing

- reconnoitring for shelter (and our existential sense of place and space and wonder)

- reading and understanding topography.

When you consider each of these tasks, you can see how the primitive drive has been usurped by the capitalist marketing machine.

- Looking for food morphs into over-eating unhealthy snacks (combining sugar, salt, and starch triggers the dopamine reward response) which can lead to obesity.

- Physiologically striving to avoid being eaten or killed engages our fight or flight response which equates with fear, which equates to at least 50 per cent of all sales pitches. All insurance is about guarding against the unknown, and the fear of what's out there that's coming to get us. (An online insurance and sales techniques guide starts with the slogan 'Fear sells, so sell fear'.)

- Bonding with the tribe becomes being sold a sense of belonging through the promise that product 'X' will make you young/wealthy/ desirable with white teeth/a gym body, etc.

- Seeking a mate – well, sex sells everything! It at least grabs our attention.

- Looking for shelter equates to finding the perfect home, taking expensive holidays, avoiding bad neighbourhoods, etc.

- The existential enquiry and sense of place transforms into wars, factions, populism, religions, and New Age beliefs, rather than an open and expansive ontological quest couched within Nature.

- Reading our topography – forget it, there's an app for that now!

Now let us reclaim and rewild our senses, starting with touch.

Touch

Four out of our five main senses are sited in the head, which appears to have some kind of hierarchical logic, and our fifth sense is touch, which we feel in our skin. Our skin is our largest organ, and largest sense organ. All of the surface of our skin is sensitive to touch, and we have varying densities of touch sensors or receptors under the skin (approximately 200 receptors per square centimetre). These are most densely concentrated in the areas of our bodies that are involved in directly exploring the environment like our hands, feet, and face. The nerve endings and pressure receptors are tactile pathways, activated through touch, which our brain uses to interpret and explore the world around us. But recent research suggests that the brain's response to touch serves an even wider purpose, providing critical stimulation during all stages of life.[141]

Our skin is the interface between our perceived internal selves and the external world (though even that is not so clearly defined as we like to think – we are permeable and leaky). Our touch receptors become stimulated and transmit messages to the brain via neurons in the nervous system. The spinal cord can also process sensory information and react in an acute or threatening situation, like pulling our hand away from a hot surface, which is a reflexive action, before the brain gets involved.

The body sends tactile information to the somatosensory cortex (represented in medical depictions as the *homunculus*, or little man) through neural pathways via the spinal cord, the brain stem, and the thalamus. The somatosensory cortex is the primary receptive area for touch sensations. Due to its many connections to other brain areas, the somatosensory cortex is the part of the nervous system that integrates touch, pressure, temperature, and pain messages.

One of the influences on the development of my work comes from *The Eyes of the Skin*, a wonderful book by the Finnish architect and philosopher Juhani Pallasmaa.[142] Pallasmaa argues for the primacy of our tactile sense, and that 'all the senses, including vision, are extensions of the tactile sense; the senses are specialisations of skin tissue, and all sensory experiences are modes of touching and thus related to tactility'.

Pallasmaa also quotes from anthropologist Ashley Montagu's assertion that:

> the skin is the oldest and most sensitive of our organs, our first medium of communication, and our most efficient protector... Even the transparent cornea of the eye is overlain by a layer of modified skin... Touch is the parent of our eyes, ears, nose, and mouth. It is the sense which became differentiated into the others, a fact that seems to be recognised in the age-old evaluation of touch as the 'Mother of all the senses'.[141]

Touch for me is related to sensuality, and sensuality flows from a total body feeling of surrender and pleasure, homecoming and juiciness. Touch is the body leading the dance with the mind. When I feel fully sensual, I can't determine which senses I am engaging, as this synaesthetic ecstasy expresses itself through my hungry, willing body in response to the multi-tactile, multi-sensuous, seductive forest: soft green ferns, wet mosses, boulders, bark, dripping leaves, humus, sunlight, water, wood, soil, dewdrops, spiders' webs, skin.

By smelling, touching, tasting, seeing, and hearing, we absorb the fecund feast of the woods in one indistinguishable relational sharing with life, one paroxysm of the desire to reinhabit our sensory beings, to re-merge with all beings in our original kinship. That's the immersion part of forest bathing – letting go and falling into the body's hands. Skin tingles, the hairs primed, we are free of restraint, free of fear, free of the illusion of a separate adult self. All body systems start a reset process, back to the individual default settings for that particular human. Carl Jung wrote, 'Matter in the wrong place is dirt, people got dirty through too much civilisation. Whenever we touch Nature, we get clean.'[143]

Is it not strange that we have to lose our self in order to find our self, that through the intervention of the inquisitive flesh, we expand beyond the illusory bounds of the skin and merge with the Mystery, the *Participation mystique*? Nan Shepherd understood this intuitively when she wrote:

> Walking thus, hour after hour, the senses keyed, one walks the flesh transparent. But no metaphor, transparent, or light as air, is adequate. The body is not made negligible, but paramount. Flesh is not annihilated but fulfilled. One is not bodiless, but essential body.[144]

Angela Carter wrote about the inherent sexual charge of the forest. In one story, she alludes to this in the title 'Penetrating to the Heart of the Forest'; in another story, the dense jungle can consume flesh, so that there is an erotic charge in this idea of metamorphosis, of therianthropy, a transformation of ingestion, decomposition, and sacramental incarnation (from *carnal* 'of the flesh'); of growing teeth and claws and becoming the jungle spirit itself, sweating and dissolving, rotting sweetly, clawing and consuming our own soft flesh, interpenetrating ourselves, merging with the green fecundity and damp mulch of her own warm flesh.

This shamanic journey is depicted in the cave art at Le Trois Freres and Lascaux, by the image of the shaman's ecstatic trance with an erection, with a bird head staff and a bison, and another image of a half person, half deer symbol of both fertility and spiritual journeying. Nature is our witness; she is our mistress too (Jung saw Nature as a female Divinity).

As therapists, we need to be comfortable in our own skin, comfortable with our own sexuality, and hold the awareness that the forest may arouse us.

In fact, if it doesn't arouse us, are we really even there, are we fully present, or are we yet again suppressing aspects of our divinity? Our clients may also experience sexual imagery and ambivalent feelings about how acceptable it is for sensuality to evoke sexuality, and feel the heightened erogenous awakening that amplifies the seduction of the forest, in arboreal and corporeal abandonment.

This can become an opportunity to explore the deeper realms of spirituality, or even open up a conversation about more practical aspects of sensuality and the subtle, constrictive censorship of society on our wild sexual power. Of course, this plays out differently with the traditional gender narratives around sexuality in our society, and what is deemed acceptable, comfortable, and compliant in our socially defined gender roles, which thankfully are now being challenged and broken down. My limited perspective would suggest that women's sexuality is something the religious male patriarchy has found quite threatening, so it has been suppressed for a long time; but it springs to life when those abstract puritanical values are shed like an unchosen skin as the path into the woods leads to the ancient worship place where all are welcome and equal.

When we make that tiny sideways step into inviting the skin to participate in our encounter with the forest, we know intuitively that we open Pandora's box of earthly delights; the whispers of the woodbine, honeysuckle, and climbing wild rose, the trembling touch, the sweet dripping liquor of the summer shower through the leaves, and we turn downwards, we go back to our own ecstatic unity with life, dropping the pretence of civility, welcoming the annihilation of self and merger with the one. This is a descendent rather than ascendent religious experience. We enter the earth; the soil is Earth's skin, so we conjoin in union.

> When the great swing has taken an individual into the world of symbolic mysteries, nothing comes of it, nothing can come of it, unless it has been associated with the earth, unless it has happened when that individual was in the body... And so individuation can only take place if you first return to the body, to your earth, only then does it become true.[145]

We get wet, we get covered in mud, we are teased by ancient ferns softly wiping our auras, we tear our clothes on brambles, we mess up our hair, we eat the fruit, we don't care; Eden is ours to reclaim. Primal skin feels alive in its own sentience, no longer a barrier, but more of an osmotic palpating portal between worlds.

A friend and I recently discussed the image I have of humans as being strange creatures without thick fur (except in a few places) we are largely naked like newborn blind rats – and she was observing how a dog expresses itself through its coat of fur, how it lies flat when the dog is calm and happy, and becomes raised when it is troubled, so it appears as if each strand of fur is like an extension of the nerve ending of the skin. Each hair could also be considered to work and coordinate collectively as the 'eyes of the skin', alert and filtering the vibrations of the air.

Maybe we still have phantom fur, our inner sense of danger causing our little hairs to rise and our skin to prick. Touch is so important to us as humans, as social mammals, that in the positive psychology construct of the Human Givens approach, touch is regarded as a form of nutrition. As Pallasmaa writes, 'The primacy of the tactile sense has become increasingly evident…the very essence of the lived experience is moulded by hapticity.'[146]

Babies of most mammals, including humans, depend on touch to thrive. The skin is our primary sense, the one that develops in the amniotic vessel of the womb at about eight weeks of gestation, and forms part of the attachment process. Some of the first touch sensors to develop are in the lips and mouth, and the oral cavity will become an important haptic sensing centre for the developing infant, mirroring the cavity of uterine development and later the creation of safe womb-like space within the home.

There is a strong identity between naked skin and the sensation of home. The experience of home is essentially an experience of intimate warmth. The space of warmth around a fireplace is the space of ultimate intimacy and comfort. Marcel Proust gives a poetic description of such a fireside space, as sensed by the skin: 'It is like an immaterial alcove, a warm cave carved into the room itself, a zone of hot weather with floating boundaries.'[147]

When I was born, the practice at the time was to remove newborns from their mothers; they would be swaddled tightly in blankets and placed in separate nurseries, only being returned to the mother at set feeding times. These separation events have a significant impact not only on the development of the newborn's neurology but also on the later sense of connection to everything and everyone beyond the perceived self. Maybe I was fortunate in that I was able to unconsciously compensate for this absence of touch by developing a deep early attachment to Nature, and maybe also in part to compensate, I am a very tactile person – I love touch, the feeling of skin on skin is sublime, a pure animal bliss, and even when I'm talking to someone, reaching out to touch or hug feels as much part of the conversation as speech.

Giving and receiving so-called pleasant touch triggers a variety of physiological responses. It reduces the cardiovascular stress response – lowering heart rate, blood pressure and the stress hormone cortisol – and triggers the brain's release of oxytocin, a neuropeptide that promotes feelings of wellbeing, devotion, and bonding.[148]

Engaging touch in the forest

Before you enter the forest, stop and stand still, feel what the body feels, extend the sense of sight into the skin only, close the eyes if it helps. What do you detect in the car park, footpath, housing estate, or wherever you are that is not forest. Feel the air around you, sense the ground, make note of all that is not-forest, and how the animal body responds, then drop it and go into the forest.

Enter and step inside a few paces, now stop and repeat this exercise. Sense the environment through the skin, touch the air, let the forest skin reach out and make contact with yours; be receptive. Your hands are great receptors for new information; feel them tingle. Stay in your body: what is around you, what is the weight of the air, its perfume, its movements, how close are the trees and how is their presentation? Feel everything swirling and pulsating like a galaxy, feel the coolness and the stillness too, as it enters into your pores, drawing toxins out and sweetening the blood.

You are now ready to explore the woods, and let them explore you in more detail. Walk in a dream, keep sight to a minimum, mostly unfocused and peripheral, and let hands, face, and bare feet (optional) explore the haptic interface and the textures of a living organism. Allow each new caress to be fully embodied in a rapturous mutual consummation. Stroke, swim, scratch, slide, smooth.

Can you feel that continuity between life expressing itself, seeking to know itself. Can you sense that you are walking on the skin of a super-organism? That you are now inside a creature? Exploring touch in the forest engages our haptic memories and serves to reignite the synaesthetic synapses. Walking gently with eyes closed or guided by a friend can be so illuminating and stimulating. One student proclaimed with joy, 'I didn't know trees had a smell'; another student had to be gently prised away from a particularly moss-covered trunk as she just wanted to cling on to its soft, nurturing 'green fur' and stay there all day.

Moving from touch to smell

From about two weeks old, a baby begins to be curious about its world and relies on the two senses of touch and smell more than the others to begin with. As it grows, the baby starts to clutch and hold things in its hands, its vision is still not yet focused fully, its hearing is working but not yet fully calibrated, and the baby is able to distinguish the prosody of the parents (have you noticed how we talk to babies in a sing-song way to demonstrate prosody, confirm that we are friend, not foe?).

Gradually, whatever is grabbed by the hands begins to make its way to the mouth, to that oral cavity, for sensing and evaluating, and as it enters the mouth and the sensitivity of the lips, it passes under the nose, where information is gathered that starts to build these maps of objects and surroundings so important for neural development. Babies can smell inside the womb, and a newborn can smell its mother from about two feet away. Taste also plays a part in this exploring-the-world process, but a newborn baby can only distinguish between sweet and sour tastes until about three months old.

Smell

Smell is such an ancient and mysterious sense, and scientists still don't fully understand how it all works, but new research indicates that quantum physics (quantum tunnelling) is implicated. In this theory, the vibrational frequencies of odorants are matched by electrons through a complex tunnelling process similar to photosynthesis.[149] We have a wide range of up to 350 different olfactory receptors that may specialise in detecting specific odours – according to a report in *Science*, humans can detect up to a trillion different odours![150]

Each odour molecule transits the nasal mucosa and binds with proteins that interact with neurons from the brain across a membrane. I like to think that when we breathe in through our nostrils, that these molecules can permeate the mucosal barrier and enter the bloodstream intact, but that is oversimplifying the process. However, volatile organic compounds (VOCs) from forest tree emissions can enter our bloodstream and affect our physiology, the small molecule size of these compounds allowing them to traverse the nasal receptor membrane. If you can smell a tree, it means some essence of that tree is inside you.

I absolutely love my sense of smell, handy if like me you have a large nose. Smells are so nostalgic, smells are evocative; they trigger memories in the brain, they take us to specific times and places if they are familiar, and they provoke curiosity if they are new and as-yet unencountered. Smells connect to feelings. Smells seem the most synaesthetic of all the senses, in that a smell will conjure an image and the feeling that follows it. Sometimes the best way to describe a smell is by a taste and vice versa – if I ask you to think of the smell of ice cream, you will probably automatically create an image of what ice cream looks like; if I ask you to think of the smell of petrol, then what happens? What comes to you when I ask you to think of the smell of rain, or an elder tree, or summer?

Urban settings can either inhibit our sense of smell or demand an involuntary reduction or physical constriction in the nasal cavity. The various different accents that are characteristic of our Northern cities in the UK are partly due to Industrial Revolution pollution levels and high rainfall, which have led to a very nasal sound in the accent, as the nose is affected by external airborne particles and smog.[151]

Our olfactory sense follows on from our kinaesthetic sense in the evolutionary hierarchy of senses. It is yet another way to read the energy of where we are and who and what we are near; it's our primitive way of gaining information about our world. Just like a snake, we can scent-map in stereo with two nostrils, so we can locate the source of a scent. Our nose opens downwards, indicating that we are swimming creatures. The very act of smelling cannot happen in a vacuum; it requires a communion with the air, and it requires an interpretation and cataloguing faculty. Our sense of smell is also closely linked to our emotion centres in the brain. Smell is phylogenetically the most ancient sense; olfaction has long been associated with primitive needs concerning reward, threat, and homeostasis.

A 2013 study looked at how our subjective sense of smell was affected by anxiety induction in human subjects, and how olfactory perception is dominated by emotion:[152]

> The olfactory sense has a unique intimacy with emotion. Unlike other senses, olfactory neuroanatomy is intertwined, via extensive reciprocal

axonal connections, with primary emotion areas including the amygdala, hippocampus, and orbito-frontal cortex.

The experiment set out to prove that by inducing an artificial anxiety state in 14 participants, there would be a measurable impact on their olfactory perceptions. They proved that high states of arousal led to an emotionally charged shift in odour perception; smells that were regarded as neutral at baseline had now become regarded as 'negative' in the tests.

I think what's useful here for us as therapists is to consider the reversal of this aetiology, so that if we take anxious people out into Nature and surround ourselves with 'natural' odours like leaf litter, damp earth, fragrance from trees and plants, animal scat, and airborne aromas, those people will inevitably become less anxious (other factors being equal like agoraphobia, hay fever, and even terrain). When we can take our participants out to the forest on a smell safari, we are in for an olfactory treat, and a tranquilising experience.

Engaging smell in the forest

As we enter the forest, our sense of smell may be slow to adjust to new surroundings, so hold back any exploration of smell until the group or individuals are ready and acclimatised. If they point out a strong or peculiar smell, you know they are ready: fox scent is good for this – it really lingers in the air, and you can tell how long ago it was there by the pungency of the aroma. If you are at the front and you come across the fox scent trail crossing the path, just stop there, don't speak, but breathe in the air and imagine the fox being there earlier, and wait for someone else to say 'What's that smell?' or to start sniffing the air. People will eventually tune their olfactory receptors in to this unmistakeable musky scent. This can then become a starting place for a conversation about smell and scent, remembering the connection to memory and emotion.

From this place, I invite participants to the 'Smell Safari'. Take off into the woods following the thread of a scent, just like a dog. Stand still, wait for something on the air, sniff in different directions, and when you pick up a scent, follow it, until you intercept another scent and follow that. The key things here are to be curious and non-judgemental of smells. All smells are welcome in this exercise with equal value worthy of curiosity. Just note how we respond to a stinking smell; notice the change to the nasal cavity.

Allow about 15–20 minutes for this and have a means of calling people back. The hope is that they will not know where they have ended up following the trail.

I love the fungus known as stinkhorn and particularly its wonderful Latin name *Phallus impudicus* – the impudent penis! In mid- to late summer in established mixed woodlands it will grow somewhere hidden away and then send out this rotting, dung-like smell to trick and attract spore-carrying flies with its sticky coating. As with most woodland scents, it travels through the air some distance, and the game is to pick up that scent and see if we can trace it back and find the brazen, erect, and stinking phallus deep in the woods.

In *Entangled Life*, Merlin Sheldrake shares a wonderful extract from Charles Darwin's grand-daughter writing about how her aunt Etty would go out each day with a hunting cloak and gloves and a special stick to seek out the stinkhorns, gather them in her basket, and return home to burn them on the fire in a locked room, such was her Victorian disgust at these impudent expressions of Nature's vitality.[153]

Taste

Taste is probably one of the least deployed of the senses within the forest environment, and our *shinrin-yoku* guided walks may be restricted for legal reasons in offering people various foraged plants. For our ancestors, taste was an extremely important aspect of forest life. With taste, we could learn about new foods and try to avoid poisonous plants and animals; people with a good sense of smell and taste were more likely to survive. In utero, babies develop tongues and taste buds early in development and are able to 'taste' what the mother has been eating, although they only have taste receptors for sweet and sour.

The physiological processes of taste and smell are both very similar in terms of the mechanics of how they work. We have taste buds in our mouth, our tongue, and our nasal cavity.[154] Remember the baby who grasps something, pulls it towards the mouth, where it goes under the nose, smell-taste-touch thus working together.

I once watched a documentary about the Baka people living in the Congo forests. They discovered a wild bee's nest very high up in a tree, so two of them climbed up, risking their lives, and cut down the hive to get the honey. There were angry bees everywhere, and people getting stung, but they had a large quantity of wild honey to share amongst the tribe. They ate some and took the rest back to share, and all the honey was eaten by the end of the day. What a treat that must have been! To suddenly have all that sugar and sweetness from all of those tropical flowers condensed into a sticky, golden feast. Hunter-gatherers don't think about saving or hoarding because they trust the forest to always provide.

Taste is about so much more than just comfort or survival, and it is probably the most culturally influenced sense globally. Sociologically, it's also interesting that we can talk about having good taste and bad taste in reference to our lifestyle choices like clothes, music, cars, partners, and jokes. Why is it connected with taste? We can also talk about an experience as having left a bad taste in the mouth, meaning something negative that lingered on after an experience, or you might say that you've developed a taste for something, referring to a new habit perhaps.

Forage

Before consuming plants, always have a good guide book with you, or someone who's knowledgeable about plants. The plants I recommend here are safe and cannot be mistaken for poisonous varieties, but you must always check and learn how to correctly identify plants through plant identification keys and specific plant features. This is a part of your background learning as a forest therapist.

It is also vital that you follow any guidelines or laws about picking flowers or plants and that you forage respectfully, leaving enough plants to breed and survive and only cropping from small areas. If in doubt, contact your local wildlife trust. Also please always ask permission from the plant before picking any parts.

If you are new to the forest but want to explore working with plant energy or foraging, a good, safe place to start is by looking for wood sorrel, *Oxalis acetosella* (there are many plants in the Oxalis family, but look specifically for wood sorrel). (The same common name may refer to a related, edible plant with a different Latin name in North America, and the plant will have yellow flowers and be slightly larger.) In the UK, wood sorrel has a delicate white flower with purple veining and grows close to the ground. It looks a bit like clover, but each leaflet of the trifolium has a heart shape, whereas clover is round. There is sometimes a pink flowered variety – a garden escape, I think. All varieties are edible.

You can find it growing in most old woods; in fact, it is an indicator for ancient woodland. It grows all year in sheltered sites and you can pick the leaves all year round – go for the young lighter green ones. Wood sorrel tastes so good; it's jam-packed with vitamin C which gives it that tangy fresh taste from the oxalic acid. It's great fresh in a salad. In my local woods, there is an Iron Age hillfort, and the wood sorrel grows around the ruins; I like to imagine the early settlers here being so grateful for the sweet, tangy taste and goodness of this little unassuming plant in early spring when nothing else was yet growing.

The other plant that I can highly recommend is wild garlic or ramsons, *Allium ursinum*. It grows in ancient woodlands that have been undisturbed for at least 100 years, and is prominent in the spring before the canopy has closed over. You will know it by the pungent aroma of the leaves and flowers. All parts are edible: the flowers taste sweet and garlicky, and in spring the leaves and flowers make a lovely wild garlic pesto. It is a blood cleanser, and is great for worming pets or humans.

Another way to engage taste is to think of all the wonderful gifts of the trees and bring some of those with you to share: pine nuts, almonds, hazel-nuts, figs, dates, carob, maple syrup – the list is endless. Offer some of your treats back to the trees to share together.

Tea ceremony

Tea ceremonies are very popular, but I am not a great fan of holding them in the woods. If I was in Japan, I would be honoured to take part in one, as it is one of the most quintessential aspects of Japanese culture; knowing the subtlety of every component and every gesture is rich with meaning, and the slow meditative silent ritual would be heaven.

However, out in the woods when we are trying to support people to engage with Nature in a non-verbal, non-intellectual way, and signpost them away from anthropocentric activity, tea ceremony feels a bit too contrived, too elaborate and leader-centred. It has a novelty appeal and it brings the group together, but it seems more focused on the needs of the participants (and/or leader for some cachet) than on trees themselves. I'd rather just come across a birch tree and browse its young spring leaves, or in winter share a bottle of sloe gin around the group and celebrate our ancient Pagan gods.

If you are intent on holding a tea ceremony, do it mindfully, plan it well, then simply pick some tips of the young shoots of trees such as Douglas fir, Scots pine, spruce, and firs. Avoid yew trees and Ponderosa and Norfolk pines. Birch leaves are a wonderful tonic, and you can even add some elder flowers. Boil up some water in the woods on an open fire or camping stove, or bring a large flask of hot water with you. Simply toss in the tree tips, etc., leave to brew for about 5–10 minutes and then serve in some small cups or glasses, and enjoy. The extent to which you make this a 'sacred' event is up to you, but if you take from the tree, please give back to the tree, at least in thanks.

On one of our courses last year, we had a participant from Hong Kong who offered to hold a tea ceremony in the woods. The beauty and the purity of it left me in tears – the student held that space so poetically, and there was a Zen-like quality to her actions and movements that was way beyond anything I could ever offer, which confirmed my decision to not do one myself. Every tiny part of the process was measured and exact and symbolic.

Smell-tasting

At our deeper level of connection, how can we find a way to actually 'taste the forest', in the way that a reptile might taste the air with its tongue? When we slow right down to tree pace, we can then begin to synaesthetically smell-taste the forest. Remember our aim is to be able to navigate through the forest guided by these two senses with our eyes closed. Hearing and touch will play their part together, but they are more our heightened, flight or fright senses, whereas smell-taste are an octave below.

The smell and taste centres in the brain are both closely linked with emotions and are a key component of our survival mechanisms. Taste is comprised not just from our taste buds, but a combination of taste, smell, temperature, and texture, and of course our anticipation/conditioning responses (Pavlovian). Taste really is about sensuality, pleasure, and arousal. Restaurants know this (well, good ones do) and exploit it to provide an all-round sensory experience, not just a palatal orgasm. Think of the craze for restaurants that serve meals in complete darkness.

When we are in the forest, how does it enhance our sensory acuity to experiment with different foods, tastes, and smells? How does an apple taste, or a mango out in the woods? Do taste and smell activate higher realms of sensory awareness when we work with a client or group together in a natural setting? What other psycho-physiological changes can we notice when we are eating in the forest?

One of the reasons why cut flowers in the house make us so happy is because our primitive brain recognises the scent of the flowers, and it knows that fruits will follow, and fruits are food. Our hunter-gatherer ancestors would follow the scent of flowers on the air, triggering the reward response in the brain, with oxytocin, dopamine and serotonin creating a heady cocktail of feel-good factors. Honeysuckle, *Lonicera periclymenum*, is a great example of a sweet-scented woodland flower growing on a climber, and you can eat the tiny centre of the flower, which is sweet, hence the honeysuckle name. Most woodland flowers try to get their business done before the canopy closes over, so you will find the best flower displays in early spring, a very tough time and harsh environment for a delicate flower to show itself – we could get hot sun one day, snow the next. They are real survivors and very hardy.

Many woodland flowers have underground bulbs or corms to store energy so they can make that early growth of reproductive parts before gaining their leaves, or losing the early weak sun to the canopy. Some of these bulbs can be dug up (check with landowners first and follow foraging guidelines) and eaten, such as pignut, *Conopodium majus*. This plant has an interesting history, and in mid-spring you will see the early typical umbellifer, deeply cut leaves, resembling the leaves of the carrot, a distant cousin. I've never found any big enough to make a meal, but they have a nice nutty taste.

Sound

For the purposes of forest bathing, I believe it is important to consider each of the senses individually and then together. Each sense offers us an insight into our evolutionary history, and our sense of hearing is a fascinating and elaborate apparatus. Although I am predominantly a visual person, I have an acute ear for music, and I love hearing our many indigenous bird songs and the messages that they convey as much as I love watching them out of the window or with my binoculars.[155]

The musician and jazz producer Joachim Ernst-Berendt (JEB) considers hearing to be our first and primary survival sense, the one we become attuned to using to sense the world from inside the womb onwards, and that the ear is the only human sense organ to perceive both numerical *quantity* and *value*.[156] In other words, we can hear notes an octave apart very accurately. JEB also feels this connection between the soul and the senses; hearing is described as a more receptive sense and sight as potentially aggressive. Hearing is more subtle, more nuanced, and even the language of sight becomes vague against the precision of the ear to discern reality. Our ears can never be closed, always open to the world.

We have two ears so we can hear in stereo, and this enables us to locate the direction of sounds. According to the National Institutes of Health:

> Our hearing involves some complex steps to convert an external noise into electrical signals in the brain.
>
> 1. Sound waves enter the outer ear and travel through a narrow passageway called the ear canal, which leads to the eardrum.
>
> 2. The eardrum vibrates from the incoming sound waves and sends these vibrations to three tiny bones in the middle ear: the malleus, incus, and stapes.
>
> 3. The bones in the middle ear amplify the vibrations and send them to the cochlea, a snail-shaped structure filled with fluid, in the inner ear. An elastic partition runs from the beginning to the end of the cochlea, splitting it into an upper and lower part. This partition is called the basilar membrane because it serves as the base, or ground floor, on which key hearing structures sit.
>
> 4. Once the vibrations cause the fluid inside the cochlea to ripple, a traveling wave forms along the basilar membrane. Hair cells, sensory cells sitting on top of the basilar membrane, ride the wave. Hair cells near the wide end of the snail-shaped cochlea detect higher-pitched sounds, and those closer to the centre detect lower-pitched sounds.
>
> 5. As the hair cells move up and down, microscopic hair-like projections (known as stereocilia) that perch on top of the hair cells bump against an overlying structure and bend. Bending causes pore-like channels, which are at the tips of the stereocilia, to open up. When that happens, chemicals rush into the cells, creating an electrical signal.
>
> 6. The auditory nerve carries this electrical signal to the brain, which turns it into a sound that we recognize and understand.[157]

All of our sensory apparatus is complex and refined, and has obviously evolved through millions of years of fine tuning. Being able to detect sound is vital to survival, for hunting food, and to avoid being hunted. Can we begin to hear again with the hunter's ears, or has our hearing atrophied as JEB suggests?[158]

It is amazing how quickly hearing can compensate when we temporarily remove sight from our range of sensing. Try just standing in the forest with your eyes closed and notice what happens, notice how hearing can almost immediately begin to compensate by building a layered sound map around you. If you gently walk towards a tree with your eyes closed, notice that you can sense when you are close to the tree; hearing and echo-location play a part in that proprioceptive sensing of ourselves in space.

Engaging auditory connection in the forest

I have developed an exercise called 'Human Radar': it takes discipline to do accurately but it is well worth persevering with. One day, I was out with students, and I would normally stay and guard their bags whilst they wander off into the woods, but on this occasion I thought I would sit down near the bags and do the exercise myself. After a few moments, I experienced the most profound shift of my assemblage point. My consciousness (my sense of me as a being) was suddenly located outside of myself and within the sounds, listening to the cross-legged me sitting in the centre; it was as if I had merged with the sounds and become identified as consciousness within them. I can't really explain, but it did show me what a powerful exercise it can be.

Leave all bags and phones, etc. at a central point and then ask participants to head off in any direction they choose. This exercise can be done walking, standing, sitting, or lying down. It can be done with eyes open or closed. Find a starting place and just remain still for a moment.

Hold your hands tightly over your ears to cut out all sounds completely for about 30–45 seconds, then put your hands down.

Now imagine that you have a series of concentric rings emanating out from your head in every direction off into the horizon.

Now, because the mind wants to be involved, see if you can hear and name each individual sound in the forest and map it on the imaginary radar, just like in films where you suddenly see or hear a blip on the ship's radar.

So, you might hear a great tit at 1 o'clock (12 o'clock tends to be straight ahead), a wood pigeon up above and at 8 o'clock, an unknown tweet-tweet bird sound at 10 o'clock, airplane directly above, insect at 3 o'clock moving to 6 o' clock on the closest ring near your head, thunder far off at 6 o'clock maybe five miles away.

Once you have expanded all the way out to the horizon, slowly bring your awareness back in again, pull those rings back all the way to about a couple of inches from your head.

Now expand out again, but this time allow yourself to hear the full orchestra, the complete symphony of the woods all in one go, the total crescendo of the sound bath. Enjoy.

I encourage you to create your own listening exercises, and you may already know another one called 'Deer Ears'. Just stand still and cup your hands around your ears as if you were forming a larger, pointy animal-type ear. Notice how it affects your hearing; try pointing one deer ear backwards, what can you hear? Although we live in an ocular-centric world, when we go into the woods, we can shift focus to our hearing sense to guide us. We can allow that rich multi-layered soundscape to dissolve into us, lifting us up and carrying us along like the pied piper, enchanted and soothed by the forest song. Closing our eyes removes the 'hegemony of vision' and allows the gentler ear to inform our sense of the world around us.

Of course, we cannot fully appreciate listening and the freshness of sound without also savouring the beauty and prescience of the original silence. Merleau-Ponty argued:

> Our view of man will remain superficial so long as we fail to go back to that origin [of silence], so long as we fail to find, beneath the chatter of words, the primordial silence, and as long as we do not describe the action which breaks this silence. The spoken word is a gesture, and its meaning, a world.[159]

This warning reminds us to place a value on silence and also to realise the power of language, and to remember the value of the unspoken gesture, the movement that spontaneously arises from the stillness and silence, the greeting of the world in all its radiant forms and expressions.

Sight

I have deliberately left our sense of sight till last, as it feels the least straightforward, passive, or innocent of all the senses. I am more drawn towards discussing sight in terms of its restriction or limitations than its presence in our perception and assimilation of our natural (forest) or urban environment. It feels that with our sight, we have this capacity for instantaneous knowledge and definition. Sight pre-empts cognition. We need to uncentre that, distract it, lead sight into unfamiliar places, and therefore gain the moment between the object and its translation.

Dominance of vision and visual bombardment

Vision and perception define and label too easily, leaving little to our unfettered imaginations, and little room for that opportunity to slip between worlds. It is a strange paradox that we need to temporarily eliminate, trick, or restrict sight in order to see. What we see with our routine, highly conditioned visual perception is largely acquisitive – we gather visual information from fixed technical parameters – but out in the forest our gaze can become more participatory, as we recalibrate vision away from definition and assumption about the nature of objects and their value, and more towards a reciprocal exploration of what phenomenologically exists. We are deceived by our mind's eye and so we miss many things, or misinterpret the energy signals of others. Some things we see that we can't comprehend, and so they become invisible; they de-exist to the mind.

Living in a predominantly ocular-centric culture can exacerbate feelings of alienation, isolation, and exteriority, and contribute to the pathology of sensory detachment and numbness. Ironically, the technology that connects people and enhances both global communication and information exchange can be part of this sense of alienation that people feel. Before mobile phones, before the PC and the internet, there was an age of greater innocence, of vagueness, and the need for concerted effort and enquiry, different modes of connection and communication.

Things were perhaps a bit dreamier, nuanced, naïve, a bit less exposed to the light of scrutiny and examination; we still had many of the same human socioeconomic problems, but our approach to life was very different. The development of mobile phone interactivity was driven by socially awkward, shy Scandinavian teenagers. Now we are all adjusted to that social behaviour pattern. The technological hegemony that translates into multichannel 24-hour TV, video games, pornography, and even social media with its narcissistic obsession with celebrity and illusion, is all predicated upon the enslavement of vision.

The more urban the setting, and the more technology we engage with, the more alienated we feel, and the more separated from our other withering senses we become. The more time we spend in *The Matrix* (Jean Baudrillard's simulacra, relating only to a facsimile of our primal home and place of belonging; see the vignette, Simulacra, following this chapter), the more we forget who and what we are. The more that we are encouraged to 'gaze', the more we become reliant on a set of predetermined Pavlovian signals that isolate and prioritise sight as the easiest instant sensory gratification dopamine hit vector. We get high and become placated/pacified by habitually reaching for visual stimulation overload, a kind of ocular-somatic opioid that has hijacked our hunter faculties. (It's funny how most of our action films still require a 'hunter' character who is hunting down a baddie, whilst being hunted themselves.)

These neural- and behaviour-changing technologies (together with the development of the application of psychology to marketing, initiated by Freud's nephew Edward Bernays) have massively influenced whole populations with visual enticement and mind control. I consider this to be what really defines the advent of the Anthropocene epoch. Michel de Certeau states: 'The current industrial mass production of visual imagery tends to alienate vision from emotional involvement and identification, and to turn imagery into a mesmerising flow without focus or participation.'[160]

Vision is the only sense to keep pace with the blurring speed of the technology. The dominance of the eye and visually engaging technologies has left us separated from life, mere spectators in an endless peep show of tragedies and doggy snacks. The commodification of visual space demands our attention, and we are bombarded with images of war and terror that eventually numb us to the shock of image and reality. From television to newspapers, from advertising to all sorts of mercantile epiphanies, our society is characterised by a cancerous growth of vision, measuring everything by its ability to show or be shown, and transmuting communication into a visual journey.[161]

Baudrillard goes as far as suggesting that the US has become one giant cinema screen. In cinema, the eye is a recurrent theme having different symbolic meanings depending on context, or sometimes left ambivalent as in Ridley Scott's iconic 1982 sci-fi film *Blade Runner*, which also reflects the legacy of the dystopian world from Orwell's *1984* and its chilling reminder that 'Big Brother is watching you', which has then ironically become a voyeuristic reality show in its own right where participants are thrown together in a house with cameras everywhere and are being watched 24 hours a day by the general population for entertainment, in a disturbing parody of our surveillance-obsessed culture, and a nod towards Jeremy Bentham's chilling Panopticon prison. Similarly, the disembodied eye features as a strange symbol in Hitchcock's 1945 film *Spellbound*. The dream sequence devised by Salvador Dali suggests that as you are looking at the screen, so the screen is looking at you, knowing your secrets, and playing on the psychological theme of this film. Sight is the only sense where the eye can see itself seeing.

There is a massive difference between adaptation and evolution, and we are still genetically and mechanically apes with big brains and opposable thumbs. Our DNA cannot keep pace with the adjustments we are required to make, as vision is co-opted into the buying and selling of goods and services using sex appeal, status, and security as common tropes for archaic social belonging/dominance needs. Children know of no other world now except the one dominated by the laptop, internet, and the video game. This is extreme excitation for the monkey mind; we are becoming stretched in a singular direction and becoming the AI that we feared would arrive, organic information processing machines conscripted into the service of what Bernays called the 'invisible government':

> The conscious and intelligent manipulation of the organised habits and opinions of the masses is an important element in democratic society. Those who manipulate this unseen mechanism of society constitute an invisible government which is the true ruling power of our country.[162]

Bernays believed that we are all driven by biological desires, urges, and instincts, and his vision was of a utopian society in which the dangerous libidinal energies that lurked just below the surface of every individual could be harnessed and channelled by a corporate elite for economic benefit. Scary stuff!

> The defensive and unfocused gaze of our time, burdened by sensory overload, may eventually open up new realms of vision and thought, freed of the implicit desire of the eye for control and power. The loss of focus can liberate the eye from its historical patriarchal domination.[163]

Seeing versus perception

Apart from birds, whose optical nerves take up a considerable portion of their brains, most animals rely more heavily on the other senses than we do, and incorporate vision into the informational matrix. Through conditioning, we have become accustomed to relying on our sense of sight as our primary information receptor for our world. In his 2005 novel *Blinding Light*, Paul Theroux writes about the central protagonist, Steadman, who becomes addicted to an Amazonian rainforest psychoactive substance that renders him temporarily blind. In his blindness, he finds that he can 'see' more clearly, and with the compensation of his other senses, he reads people and their motives from subtle clues in their bodies that he was totally unaware of when he had full vision. He can literally smell people's feeling states.

I feel that this is a useful analogy for us when we enter the forest. If we can close our eyes and feel into the forest, we learn so much more than our eyes are accustomed to showing us. Our eyes are hard-trained to modernity, and in order to effectively unlock full-spectrum seeing and perception, we need to retrain the eyes and the mind from their habitual, preconditioned states.

This numbing down or blunting of the senses is often defined as sensory adaptation, and from an ontological perspective it is seen as an evolutionary function to decrease sensitivity in an organism to continued stimulation. Its purpose is to remove sensory data passing to the brain which concerns unchanging or constant environmental conditions, thereby allowing the brain to be focused on any changes to conditions which could give the organism an adaptive advantage. Our perception is keyed in to notice changes to the environmental background. I am thinking of how this might affect a person biologically when subjected to an urban environment over a considerable period of time, where there may be a daily routine but also an overwhelming amount of stimulus, which could cause a sensory shutdown.

In the work of Kaplan and Kaplan,[164] when examining the visual-neural benefits of being in Nature in what they term 'restorative environments', they discuss how the eyes convey information to the brain that allows for cognitive de-stressing and neural 'de-fragging' to occur. De-stimulating or consciously withdrawing sight gives the brain less stimulus and also permits the process of restoration and neural housework to take place. We know this from sleep, meditation, and simply being (safely) in the dark. We slow down. Due to their disproportionately larger visual cortex, birds of prey respond to having a hood put over their heads by just becoming calm; if they can't see, they don't exist, they just switch off.

Each sense acts as an energy transducer and each is equivalent but different in how it apprehends an object. If I hold an apple in my hand with my eyes open, my brain can identify it as apple in a nanosecond, so the other senses feel redundant – 'OK, well, you don't need us anymore, job done, but just to back up that label, I'll have a little sniff, and I'll feel the weight and texture of the apple in my hand.' Now close your eyes and let someone place a fruit in your hand. The other senses, the neglected senses, are now doing what they were honed to do, reading the object through haptic qualities, smell, weight and texture. We can't see the other side of an object such as an apple, so we can't get a three-dimensional sense of the apple until it is in our hands or touching our skin. Try it out.

Allowing the other senses to work as a team without a dominant boss creates greater synergy and therefore opens up sensing pathways closer to unconscious perception than conscious reasoning. Remember we are trying to 'see' the world as it is, not how we are trained/habituated to perceive it.

The writer Aldous Huxley suffered from congenital sight problems, and as well as his novel *Eyeless in Gaza*, he wrote a book called *The Art of Seeing* about his experiences of attempting to improve his eyesight based on the Bates Method, which combines eye exercises with an understanding of the psychological influence of the mind on sight. He describes the process of seeing broken down into three subsidiary processes: sensing, selecting, and perceiving.

- Sensing: the raw material of seeing, the *sensa* which occur within the total visual field, that which can be sensed in any given moment.

- Selecting: the process of filtering which follows sensing. A part of the visual field is selected, singled out from the rest. The clearest image is at the central point of the retina. We choose our focus, a phylogenetic survival development: directed attention, or as Huxley refers to it, voluntary attention.

- Perceiving: the final part of the process in which the selected object or sensa is identified by the brain. The sensa are interpreted by the mind as the appearance of a physical object in space.[165]

I'm sure that Huxley's life and writing (he had a colleague called Steedman) was a major influence on Theroux's book, alongside the writings of William Burroughs. Like Theroux's protagonist Steadman, Huxley also had a life devoted to experimenting with the effects of psychoactive substances on his consciousness, and how his perception fields were broadened and shifted out of the comfortable, mundane associations and into realms of vision beyond ordinary reality. He described his experiences with mescaline in his seminal work *Doors of Perception*, the title taken from a quote by another visionary, William Blake:

> If the doors of perception were cleansed every thing would appear to man as it is: Infinite. For man has closed himself up, till he sees all things thro' narrow chinks of his cavern.[166]

I suspect that Huxley with his limited eyesight became engrossed with the idea of experiencing the kinds of angelic and beatific visions achieved naturally and spontaneously by Blake, and in mescaline he saw an opportunity to reach the 'sacramental vision' he sought. Mescaline is renowned for producing bright colourful visions and these are projected on to the inner eye. Huxley recorded in *Doors of Perception* that he only saw lights and shapes, not the extra-ordinary states of mind and the visionary landscapes he sought, but later in life he realised that these images were just temptations that were keeping him from the true realisation of the unity of the cosmos. In a letter to Dr Humphry Osmond in 1955, he describes an attempt under the guidance of his partner Laura to use mescaline to access early childhood memories, but instead:

> what came through the closed door was the realisation – not the knowledge, for this wasn't verbal or abstract – but the direct, total awareness from the inside, so to say, of Love as the primary and fundamental cosmic fact... I was this fact; or perhaps it would be more accurate to say that this fact occupied the place where I had been.[167]

This is a great parallel for the therapeutic process that can take place in the forest. Closing our eyes can induce feelings of vulnerability and disorientation. I prefer closed eyes to blindfolds as this gives the participant full ownership of the exercise and allows them to be fully sighted again in an instant, whereas a blindfold is an imposition, a material shackle to vision. What we are looking for is to invite that vulnerability and disorientation but in a way that puts the participant in full control so that if they feel overwhelmed, they can open the eyes.

I have occasionally experienced this sense of ego annihilation in Nature that Huxley writes about, but it is an elusive event which seems to happen spontaneously of its own accord, and I have yet to understand how to engage it voluntarily just from being in Nature, but then maybe that's the ego looking to regain control, which is a paradox. This state of oneness is open to all people and it resides very close to the path of ordinary consciousness, accessible to anyone. It is not something that requires years of study, or meditation or fancy breathing. It's just about finding or being led to the door, and stepping through. The only preparation that I can elicit so far is to be child-like and playful – that is, to just turn up as yourself, no preparation, intellectualisation, or preconception. No agenda.

There are many ways to explore our other senses in Nature, and to remain unsighted can create profound insights. It's amazing how quickly our other senses become more engaged once 'the hegemony of vision'[168] has been neutralised. Sight is literal; other senses are more nuanced, more reciprocal. In medieval times, it was believed that when you looked at something, an invisible thread left your eye, literally an eye-beam, and then returned with an imprint of the object; hence the lines from 'The Extasie', a poem by the metaphysical poet John Donne in 1633:

Our eye-beams twisted, and did thread
Our eyes upon one double string

This was known as the Emission theory[169] and gradually became replaced with the more popular Intromission theory which postulates that visual perception is obtained by light coming from the object entering the eyes. Modern science has demonstrated that we see a representation of that object which is physically transmitted by photons from a light source, such as the sun, to visible objects, and finally passing through a lens, such as a human eye or camera. The object appears upside down and so the brain reverses the image so it appears as it is.[170]

We need to be careful to differentiate between visual perception and mental perception, and understand how sight both affects perception and how it can deceive it. Is perception active or passive? And is perception selective based on genetic, social, cultural, and environmental factors? I might see a beautiful oak tree, another may see a source of timber and income, another may regard the tree with fear or disdain and think it should be felled because the leaves are blowing into their gutter, yet another may see a place to climb, or want to make a painting of the tree, for another it may serve as a reminder of the tree that their partner hanged themselves from some time ago. The oak tree remains the same.

If I keep going back to visit this tree on a long and regular basis, my perception of this oak will change too; my appreciation of its beauty and the characters of oak will be enhanced as I get to feel and understand its personality. I may project or transfer feelings and associations on to the oak tree, I may come to regard it as 'my tree' and become possessive towards it, or I may come and just listen to this wise, old being who has withstood all the vagaries of time and weather and change, and I might reflect on the impermanence of life and how transitory everything is, and that might cause me to let go of the clinging places.

It is way beyond the scope of this book to delve deeper and wider into the fascinating topic of perception and some of the philosophical arguments around it. I direct the reader towards the work of Maurice Merleau-Ponty and his work on the phenomenology of perception. Merleau-Ponty argues that there is a unity of body and sensory experience, that we as sensing beings are not separate from that which we are sensing; we live in a participatory Universe:

> The world is...the natural setting of, and field for, all my thoughts and all my explicit perceptions. Truth does not inhabit only the inner man, or more accurately, there is no inner man, man is in the world, and only in the world does he know himself.[171]

Jung was also curious about perception and distinguished between perception as sensation, the psychological function that can perceive the immediate environment through the bodily senses, and perception as intuition, the psychic function that perceives possibilities largely through the unconscious. Intuition gives outlook and insight; it revels in the garden of magical possibilities as if they were real.[172] (For more on intuition and instincts from Jung's perspective, see 'Intuition' in Chapter 13, The Savage Self.)

However, it is important to realise or bring into our conscious awareness how and why we perceive, the limits of perception, the combinations of sensory inputs that shape our worlds, and how perception is also dependent on knowledge and context. I am interested in how our perception tricks us and how we can trick our perception, so that we can explore the hidden fabric of the Universe, how we can get back to child-like states of consciousness. Jung regarded both sensation and intuition as irrational functions, meaning arbitrary. He understood the imperative of finding our way back to precognitive states in Nature, and in our forest bathing practice we can concern ourselves with shifting perception towards archaic sensing and away from habitual anthropomorphising and consensual familiarity.

I remember an occasion back in my student days when I was walking home from the pub at night, and I passed a house with a small front garden with a railing fence at the front. As I walked past, and in a particular light, whether moon or streetlight, out of the corner of my eye, I became transfixed by a dancing snake. I couldn't look directly at it because I was immobilised, and scared it would hypnotise me, I couldn't move from the spot and escape.

I was quite literally frozen in some very ancient survival mechanism, unable to move, with this snake weaving and dancing in the corner of the garden.

Luckily a friend came along and helped me to turn round and see that it was a fern frond that was just catching a slight breeze and moving hypnotically in the semi-darkness. My terror immediately dropped away, and the spell was broken. My perception had caught something without seeing it fully and had retrieved an ancient memory from my databanks, a Universal and archetypal fear, but not the reality of my environment; I know British snakes don't rear up like a cobra, and generally never go around at night, but my logical brain was unavailable to me in this context. A fascinating experience.

So finally to the exercises: let's start small and build up our sensory muscles.

Perhaps try this exercise standing up; if you like you, can hold on to a tree or a branch. Just stand there, close the eyes and allow the senses to fill the space around you and create an internal picture of your world; be strong and still. If these exercises out in wild Nature feel too strong to start with, then try doing this on your veranda, or sitting in your garden, or even in your car with the door or windows open. It's important to start where you feel safe and strong and build from there.

Once you are happy standing with your eyes closed, the next big step is to try to walk with eyes closed. This is actually easier than it might sound once we are tuned in to this mode of being; we can see in darkness.

It's a bit like having those lines down the side that fish have to navigate by (lateral line organ). You begin to just sense your environment. It does take time to get it, so be patient and obviously start somewhere safe with no obstacles to trip over. Just walk a few paces, stop, breathe, then go again; stop when you begin to feel unsure and just ground yourself. Set off again and repeat.

If you feel wobbly, just stop and go back to your anchor: your feet on the earth, your legs slightly bent; feel the core of you, and when you move forward, move with purpose, stay grounded, let your animal self take over for you and guide you. Trust that vestibular sense that keeps you upright; trust your proprioception that orients you in space. Maybe choose a tree ahead and walk towards it – feel your way there by connecting to the tree and being reeled in. Go slow and feel your way.

Finally repeat the walking part but this time with bare feet. Some of you might find this easier; just try to avoid areas where you know there will be brambles and sharp spiky twigs on the ground, or biting things. Moss and leaves and mud are great. If you feel really bold, try this exercise in a small stream, allowing your bare feet to now become the eyes. Barefoot with eyes closed is a real meditation on awareness, trust, and balance; feeling the ground, reading its sensual curves and undulations. It calls back to mind Pallasmaa's wonderful book *The Eyes of the Skin*.

Take yourself out into nature somewhere where you won't be disturbed; go to the loo first, and make sure you are warm enough and hydrated. Take something to sit or lie on.

Let the place find you. Sit or lie down if you live in a part of the world where doing that is possible without being bitten. Once you have got yourself comfortable, just close your eyes and go within. That means shutting down our main threat alert system, the eyes, and just sitting or lying still. Don't set a time limit please, don't try to breathe in any particular way, don't try to visualise anything or anyone – just be.

Keep it very simple and clear. Feel the darkness of your eyes closed, but again don't focus on anything; just settle into place and let whatever comes happen around you. If you sense something or someone in your field, open your eyes, be alert but still. Remain with your self. Once you settle, you will slow right down and then those compensating senses will be switched on, reading your environment in 360 degrees. Just stay there until it feels complete, this sensing process in calmness. If you fall asleep, all the better – I have had many clients fall into a deep slumber after these exercises.

Simulacra

Writing a book about Nature is totally impossible – bugs crawl across my page, a moth flies around the room, a fir cone looks at me longing for my touch, blue tits peck at my windowpanes, and now, after the rain, John Donne's 'Busy old fool, unruly Sun' has come out to tempt me yonder. How does anyone ever get any writing done?

We cannot ever convey the immediate three-dimensional 'everything everywhere all at once' nature of experience, so we end up writing a book about our interpretation of Nature, and our descriptions are relative to our own understandings, personal filters, colonial/Christian and anthropocentric discourses, cultural affiliations, mythologies, and relationships with Nature, which includes the inner nature in various ecologies.

In order to attempt to convey this subtle incomprehensible force, artists paint not the landscape but the mood and the feeling of the landscape, likewise in photography and music. In prose, the written word, we resort to language, and language is both limited and loaded; the complex essence of the multidimensional, multirelational reality of Nature gets lost in the static of words. Language imprisons and relativises the aliveness of pre-agricultural or Palaeolithic experiences within us – try explaining a dream that leaves you feeling unsettled or elated. Our peak mystical experiences are ineffable, therefore unspeakable; it can be frustrating, but maybe just to have the feelings and the memories is sufficient.

We filter those experiences through the lenses of education, need for societal approval, and moral and religious paradigms that may still reflect earlier prejudices and negative biases towards Nature, and that shift from trust to acquisition and wealth/fear.

A book on Nature therefore suffers the dilemma of wanting to educate or convey feelings about Nature, but inevitably becomes an accumulative contribution of what French Philosopher Jean Baudrillard describes as a simulacrum – a representation or imitation of something that may no longer even exist, but which becomes a kind of definitive of that reality, a symbol of a culturally constructed reality, that generation after generation grows further and further away from the original truth, and further invested in the illusion. Ultimately, simulacra point to the fact that that reality never existed, or even that nothing ever existed.

Baudrillard argues 'that society has replaced all our reality with symbols and signs, and that human experience is a simulation of reality'.[173] Why do I keep thinking of *The Matrix* when I am writing this? Maybe because the Wachowskis used this premise when they wrote the script for the film. Eventually, we succumb to the simulation of reality, and the simulacra replace all meaning and understanding in our lives. Baudrillard believed that this saturation with symbols that replace genuine experience eventually leads to a sense of total meaninglessness. TV, video games, VR headsets, Disneyworld, supermarket food, fast food, etc.

So why, then am I attempting to write not just a book about Nature but a complex interrogation of our relationship with Nature and where it deviated? It feels vital that we don't just rely on another's words or experiences to vicariously live out our sense of connection, and so, if anything, my hope is that these words may provoke some of you to go and spend more time in Nature with a new perspective, an open countenance, or a renewed appreciation for the natural world and how it interferes with our feverish pre-occupations, as she attempts to seduce us away, a sprite or a siren or some other mythical enchantress, enticing us away from our 'grown-up' pursuits, to come and play.

I refuse to accept the fugazi, the illusory nature of the simulacra; I don't want to lose my sense of connection to the earth and to know what is real, what exists eternally, and irrevocably beyond the confines of social mores, what makes me feel truly alive – that is what I'm curious about. The other side of that equation is to discuss how our socially constructed human-primate lives fit within these existential constructs and this ontological curiosity. I reject the simulacra, and choose to come back into my heart, swim naked in the cold river, and become aware as much as possible.

CHAPTER 11

Phytoncides and Trees

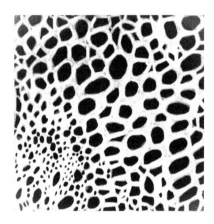

Phytoncide means 'exterminated by the plant', and the term was first coined by Russian biochemist Dr Boris Tokin from Leningrad University in 1928. Tokin was experimenting with plants to understand how they protected themselves from attack by insects and herbivores, and fungal attack (rotting). (I sense that Tomohide Akiyama from the Japanese Ministry of Agriculture was well aware of this body of research into phytoncides when he first proposed the creation of the *shinrin-yoku* walks in 1982 in Japan.)

Phytoncides are volatile organic compounds (VOCs) released by all plants as a biological defence mechanism against attack, producing a familiar pungent scent, most noticeably exuded by conifers. VOCs are made up of individual terpenes, the variety and number of which could be in the thousands. These terpenes are combined into different cocktails to the advantage of the plant in its defence mechanisms. Some of the major terpenes found in conifers and other plants are limonene, pinene, and myrcene, which give off that lovely piney, lemony Christmas tree scent. VOCs are released by trees into the atmosphere as aerosols, which we breathe in when we walk in the forest. It is these potent phytoncide compounds that are the pharmacologically active component of the forest bathing experience.

Phytoncide release into the air has seasonal diurnal cycle variations and is highest around 30°C. For example, in the Blue Mountains above Sydney, Australia, the eucalyptus trees release their pollen in what seems like a coordinated response, and leads to a dense blue cloud of pollen and VOCs – hence the name Blue Mountains.[174, 175] Some inconclusive research has suggested that trees can coordinate the release of phytoncides and pollen (known as masting) to contribute towards 'cloud seeding' to deliberately control the weather, and current research has indicated that pollen and VOCs (terpenes) now play a significant role in cloud formation.[176]

VOCs and health
Immunity

There is now a burgeoning body of evidence from Japan and elsewhere from the last 30 years to support our understanding of how these volatile oils emitted by trees have a positive immunological impact on humans. Researchers like Dr Miyazaki and Dr Qing Li have conducted numerous experiments and clinical trials with far-reaching health consequences.[177] One of the key findings of their research is that time spent in the forest is proven to increase the activity and number of NK (natural killer) cells in the body, and intracellular anti-cancer proteins. These specialised T cells or T lymphocyte NK cells, alongside T cells, are part of the body's adaptive immune response to specific pathogens, and are responsible for targeting cancerous or virally damaged and diseased cells for termination.

Research findings have indicated that NK cell counts can remain elevated for seven days to one month after just one full day spent in the forest on a *shinrin-yoku* walk. What this means in effect is that one day a month spent hanging out in the forest is sufficient to increase the efficiency of our depleted immune systems for up to a month – imagine that as a doctor's prescription! I find this an absolute miracle. Also, it's not a coincidence that the defence mechanisms a tree has evolved to protect itself from attack has this protective effect on humans; we evolved within the forest environment over many millions of years. We share an average of 15 per cent of our DNA with all trees, but perversely that number jumps to 60 per cent with banana trees. We are closely related.

When you analyse the properties of the essential oils distilled from tree resins, you begin to realise the amazing natural pharmacy in the forest that we had forgotten, and only now are beginning to fully understand and appreciate. For example, yuzu oil can be used as an antibacterial, antidepressant, antiseptic, antispasmodic, antiviral, carminative, digestive stimulant, expectorant, sedative, stomachic, anti-inflammatory, rejuvenating skin treatment, anti-oxidant, and for liver detox.

Stress

The heady bouquet of spicy scents we smell in a forest is made up of the VOCs from different trees mixing together and creating an air bath of calming, sedating, detoxifying, and healing chemicals. Many of these terpenoids have a powerful effect on the brain, acting almost like a narcotic by tranquilising and soothing the neural receptors that have been triggered by stress.[178] For example:

- Limonene is an antidepressant and anxiolytic. It reduces depression via the 5HT pathway, and stress, anxiety, and insomnia by activating adenosine receptors in cell membranes, improving nerve function and dopamine transmission. Limonene is implicated as a key factor in aerosol formation as a carrier for other terpenes, and is the most widely researched of the tree terpenes.

- Myrcene is one of the major oils found in plants and is an active constituent of cannabis, and contributes to its particular aroma, but it is also common in many other plants and trees and has a predominantly sedating and pain-relieving (analgesic) effect.

- Pinene has also been widely researched:

    A wide range of pharmacological activities have been reported, including antibiotic resistance modulation, anticoagulant, antitumor, antimicrobial, antimalarial, antioxidant, anti-inflammatory, and analgesic effects. The most prominent effects of α- and β-pinene, comprise their cytogenetic, gastroprotective, anxiolytic, cytoprotective, anticonvulsant, and neuroprotective effects, as well as their effects against oxidative stress, pancreatitis, stress-stimulated hyperthermia, and pulpal pain.[179]

It has been calculated that trees emit an approximately 1 billion tonnes of VOCs as bio-aerosols per annum into the Earth's atmosphere, 80 per cent coming from the last remaining 18 per cent of rainforest.[180] In atmospheric processes, bio-aerosols play a key role in the formation of cloud droplets, ice crystals, and precipitation, and, in combination with forests, can have significant impact on the hydrological cycle as well as atmospheric chemical composition and physics. Plant pollen, fungal spores, bacteria, algae, and cyanobacteria have been identified in bio-aerosol samples.

Stress is now a global epidemic and goes hand in hand with our modern industrial lifestyles. As a species, we evolved perfect biochemical responses to handle short-term acute stress; when that stress becomes an insidious, chronic maladjustment to life, our bodies keep deploying systems that were designed only to be used temporarily to maximise our survival mechanisms – fight, flight or freeze – resulting in an unsustainable elevation of adrenaline, cortisol, and testosterone. We were never designed to maintain these elevated states, and whilst in short-term acute incidents they do no harm, over periods of time the redistribution of energy and resources into those physiological responses depletes all of our health-enhancing rest, restore, and digest processes (parasympathetic) that affect gut health, cell growth, healing, immune function, and recovery.

The healing, tranquilising, and adaptogenic properties of phytoncides and essential oils as aerosols in the atmosphere can help to mitigate against stress factors. The combination of the various components of forest bathing is one potential antidote to stress, and this has been a key driver in the origin and promotion of forest bathing in Japan and South Korea.

Other effects on human health

We are only beginning to see the impact on human viability of our deficient, tired immune systems combined with the depletion of our natural health support resources (trees, plants, water, air, quality food, contemplation). The prevalence of new diseases that have 'jumped across' from animal species to humans should concern us. Since the 1940s and the intensification of agriculture, some 300 new infectious diseases have arisen, e.g., HIV, Zika, Ebola, SARS, MERS, and new strains of birdflu. There is little doubt about the origins of these new illnesses and pandemics.

Human populations are spilling over into deforested areas, and displaced, highly stressed animals are in close contact with people and their livestock (such as the bats in Wuhan?), leading to cross-contamination with previously unencountered germs and microbes. Industrialised agriculture and soils depleted of nutrients, coupled with an obsessive compulsion with cleanliness and pill-taking, weaken already chronically overloaded immune systems, which means we need all the 'natural' support our bodies can get to resist infections.

We have yet to fully understand the complexity of forest ecology, the symbiotic relationships that specific trees have with each other, the quantum mechanics involved in photosynthesis processes,[181] soil ecology, and the complex relationships between trees, soil, and the mycorrhizal fungal networks that connect them, and how their combined biogenic contributions to the atmosphere impact on human health, but I would suggest that without breathing in those microdoses of VOCs, we would all suffer far greater bacterial and viral infections.

Think of it this way: our immune systems evolved in symbiosis with our Earth through the soupy VOC-laden pre-industrial atmosphere. Terpenes are largely oil soluble, and apart from breathing them in, we also readily absorb them through our pores and into the adipose layers of the skin, which increases a metabolic stimulating hormone, adiponectin. We are dependent on our environments and biosphere in so many interconnected and holistic ways.

A report released in 2020 indicates that regions of Italy with a higher percentage of Mediterranean plant cover led to greater degrees of immunoprotection from COVID-19.[182] We know how pungent and aromatic the herbs and trees of this area can be. The herbs of the 'maquis' are well known for their healing and culinary uses (many traditional Italian cheeses were rolled in herb combinations due to their antibacterial and antifungal properties). Laurel bay has strong antiviral properties, and higher concentrations of native *Laurus nobilis* correlated with a lower incidence of SARS-CoV-2 infections.

We need trees more than we think, especially as climate change means more favourable conditions for the proliferation of airborne diseases, and particulate matter pollution now responsible for many deaths worldwide. Trees mitigate airborne pollution by absorbing particulate matter and releasing oxygen alongside phytoncides. In addition, phytoncides have demonstrated capacities for:

- wound healing
- reducing cholesterol and weight
- relieving depression
- reducing blood pressure
- enhancing sleep
- improving memory, perception, and cognitive learning
- enhancing antibiotic activity
- increasing respiratory capacity
- reducing shock, pain, and inflammation.

I strongly recommend that you explore the essential oils that come from trees, particularly the sacred trees of Japan, alongside camphor, yuzu, and the combined effects of frankincense and myrrh, which has attracted some interesting research.

Choose high-quality oils and put them in a diffuser, or mix with a carrier oil for a hot bath. Very few oils are toxic to the skin, but always check first if you are sensitive to them. I take essential oils out into the woods with me and then share them at the end of the session sometimes. I also use them to ward off colds and viruses, and for other health needs. They are completely amazing.

Resilience?

Resilience is a word that I feel quite ambivalent about. Four years ago, I was asked to be a part of a small group set up to essentially patch people up emotionally who had come back from the frontline of activism and protest. Of course, I immediately thought of the forest and the moor as a place for healing and recentring, but I felt uneasy about just using Nature, and this term resilience that everyone was bandying about. It felt like we were saying that if we give these people some care, they can go back to the front and get even more destroyed. It didn't feel kind or sensible, or, dare I say it, natural. Resilience felt like applying ever thicker layers of emotional and mental armour for protection, plastering over the cracks. People who stand up for the planet are modern-day heroes, and we do need direct-action activism (of that I am convinced), but at what sacrifice to our health?

Forest bathing in its purest form as practised in Japan also feels like a way to soothe nerves and decrease heart rates and blood pressures in order to carry on doing the same things that ultimately also may cause the destruction of Nature. It doesn't seem to make sense, and it also feels like another example of treating Nature as a free and disposable resource. Of course, the forests may still remain as a result of these forest therapy stations in Japan, but somehow there feels like a disconnect, using Nature objectively as a resource to ameliorate the effects of urban life, in order to go back and do more of the same.

Surely, it is far better to integrate Nature into our lives, to decrease production, consumption, working hours, and health bills to improve the overall health of the nation. Japan has so many old crafts and the connection to a slower organic, earthy and mindful lifestyle is nearer the surface than in most industrialised cultures. It's disingenuous to just spend time in the forest for a reset, getting your physiological markers recorded to indicate that your pulse rate has dropped, and then hammering the body even more (and also tending to ignore lifestyle factors within this equation, it becomes yet more abuse of

Nature, and self). Being congruous with Nature means being vulnerable and strong equally, learning from the many beings whose resilience and stamina can also be very quickly compromised by our artificial interventions.

I'm keen to see Deep Forest Bathing being offered where people are encouraged to offer a day of their week to care for and be with Nature and bring that nature-connection into their homes, habits, and personal 'gestalts'. Forest medicine has much to offer, and we can learn new ways to respect these gifts by living complementary lives, sacrificing monetary wealth for holistic ecosophic wealth. Ironically, getting back to Aristotle's idea of 'Eudaemonia' – of finding happiness in virtue and living life according to one's true spirit – may actually lead to greater performance, improve productivity, and lessen costs due to ill health.

CHAPTER 12

Risk

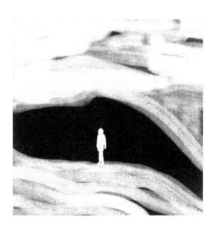

Security is mostly a superstition. It does not exist in nature, nor do the children of men as a whole experience it. Avoiding danger is no safer in the long run than outright exposure. Life is either a daring adventure or nothing.

HELEN KELLER[183]

Health and safety, and risk assessment

The subject of risk comes up frequently in conversation with colleagues, students, and commissioners, and it is important to clarify the position with regard to risk and risk management. Living in a Western high-income nation, we expect that certain things have been risk-assessed and that someone somewhere has checked that things are safe for us to use, such as trains, planes, ferries, football stadiums, public and private buildings, and even the pavements we walk on. And yet all of these have seen some of the worst civil accidents in our history: trains crash, planes crash (not very often), ferries

186

sink, stadiums collapse or people are crushed (see the Hillsborough Disaster of 1989, or the 2022 AFCON football game in Cameroon).

We can trip over hazards and bang our heads on things from time to time, but we tend to assume that our safety has vicariously been taken care of, and that we don't need to be constantly alert to danger. Of course, in many low-income countries, safety measures may be less stringent or non-existent, and so people adapt to that particular level of public and personal risk and safety. And yes, there are far more fatalities from car accidents in these countries, but statistics don't convey the whole picture.

We have a relationship to risk that assumes a certain level of care, and that health and safety regulations are in place. This is a good thing and has saved many lives, but as we see from the above examples, and many more like the 2017 Grenfell Tower fire in London (when 72 people died in an inferno as a result of non-fireproof exterior cladding having been used), we cannot always trust that safety protocols have been adhered to, or that they existed in the first place.

Health and safety laws exist to establish legal safety and quality frameworks for the protection of both members of the public and workforce from accident and injury. They create a chain of responsibility and accountability, alongside a set of agreed measures, reporting and monitoring structures, and identified liabilities. This is very important because we can't spend our time checking every single environment that we encounter in our lives – we come to expect a certain standard.

We transfer or entrust that risk assessment process to others on our behalf. In that sense, we abdicate responsibility for our safety based on assumptions commonly held about our environment within society. Our perception that we are safe is never challenged until something happens. In some countries, people are more alert to the sounds of gunfire, the threat of earthquakes, storms, wildfires, avalanches, volcanos erupting and many other natural and human threats to survival. In some ways, we adjust to these impending conditions and circumstances. We adapt and normalise risk.

Alongside this, we live in a world where we are constantly being bombarded with a narrative of fear, and messages about how unsafe everything is; about how we are under threat from all sides, how we need to get insurance for every sort of issue we can imagine, and finally, when things go wrong, who we can blame, punish, or litigate against. This all-pervading narrative attempts to prime us for imminent attack and harm, and succeeds in making us wary, anxious, on edge and risk-averse. People in urban economies are becoming more and more anxious each year.

There are very strict rules governing outdoor activity providers, and it's mandatory for staff to be fully trained and have completed the relevant qualifications and safety assessments for equipment, methods, and venues. As a qualified outdoor instructor myself, I am so glad that these legal standards exist, having been around at the time of the Lyme Bay tragedy in 1993 where four children drowned due to a lack of adequate qualified supervision.

As forest bathing walk leaders, it is also necessary that we conduct rigorous risk assessments of the sites that we intend to visit, listing all the possible risks and dangers, and then recording what steps we have taken to minimise or mitigate against those hazards or risks like slips, trips, falls, and falling branches. We also need to risk-assess the individuals in our groups that we lead in the woods, and this can be problematic, particularly if they are unknown members of the public turning up for an event, and we have not had contact with them beforehand. Do we send out a form requesting information? Are we likely to get one returned and will it be accurate? How do we turn someone away? We are in a logistic and moral dilemma.

I have developed a method of risk assessment which has served me well for the last 30 years and has never failed. It's probably something you do unconsciously already, and it involves our friend the vagus nerve. When each person arrives for a session, I make sure that I shake their hand and look them in the eyes, and that's my risk assessment right there in that moment done. That sensory contact, even though brief, tells me all I need to know about the person. My vagus nerve, my hippocampus and amygdala, and my gut instinct take milliseconds to assess the person based on those two points of contact: the hand and the eye. We can instantly process information and, 'unconsciously comprehend what it is, decide whether we like it or not; the "cognitive unconscious" presents our awareness with not just the identity of what we see, but an opinion about it.'[184]

I have learnt to filter for what I need to know: is it safe to be in a remote location with this person? If I intuitively feel unsure, then I will keep an eye on the person and see how they interact socially before we set off, and will monitor them whilst we are on the walk. If I'm still not sure, or my instinct is alerting me, I will sidle up next to them and have a little chat whilst we are walking, to ascertain, for example, whether they just had a big row before they arrived or received some bad news, or are just feeling a bit rough today. I might then advise them to just relax and enjoy being with the trees. It's my animal sense that needs to feel secure and content with someone when I'm in the woods, and once you get attuned, it's fairly clear when something doesn't feel right.

Risk aversion versus risk engagement

By avoiding risk and by fearing the journey, we are not really alive. Our bodies and our beings are beautifully and perfectly designed for risk; it's hardwired into our DNA. Risk was a daily reality of our ancestors' existence, and engaging with risk and with danger is what switches on all of our senses and brings us to the edgespace. Because in Westernised societies food and water are now largely available, we have turned our attention away from survival needs towards material goals and status concerns, which in turn has led to an increase in generalised anxiety disorders and narcissism. As risk is an inherent part of survival activities, it is by returning to more familiar hunter-gatherer environments that we can pacify the anxiety that leads to risk aversion, which in turn leads to greater alienation and then greater anxiety.

There is a big difference between human- or urban-based and Nature-based hazards. There is also a big difference between engaging with risk and being reckless or foolhardy. In our urban domesticated surroundings, we surrender the need to be fully awake to our environment, but out in the wild, we need to have everything switched on, we need to be fully present in the moment in our bodies. Warwick Cairns has written an excellent book on this topic called *How to Live Dangerously: Why We Should All Stop Worrying, and Start Living*. Warwick takes a very pragmatic approach to this topic and in his introduction suggests that when we stop worrying and live a bit more, we take more risks, and that bad things will happen but many more good things will also happen, things that will 'make you feel intensely and passionately alive'.[185] I thoroughly agree with this sentiment and I think that it's risk taking that keeps us young, and conversely risk aversion is a form of death.

In UK forests, probably the biggest threat is from other *Homo sapiens*, followed by their dogs, and cattle. Trees account for about six deaths per year in the UK (or about 1 in 10 million) and the majority of those occur in urban settings and during high winds.[186] The figure is approximately 100 per year in the US, but this figure also includes industry accidents.

Managing risk: a conjuring act

We need to feel comfortable with risk in our own lives and in natural environments, and have that balance between caution and adventure. Risk awareness is largely down to: experience + knowledge + instinct + time = wisdom. I will discuss more about what that risk might constitute in this particular setting and discipline, but initially I'll explore how and why we manage risk based on work coming from Mountain Leadership theories.

Real risk or real danger is avoided; however, a client's subjective experience of perceived risk aims to guide them just outside of their comfort zone. Colin Mortlock defines four stages of play:

- Stage 1: Play – characterised by little emotion through relatively easy participation in activities that are below the person's skill level.

- Stage 2: Adventure – characterised by enjoyment and excitement, where a person is using their capabilities more fully but maintains control over themselves.

- Stage 3: Frontier Adventure – characterised by peak experience which emerges from a person experiencing adventurous challenges very close to their limits.

- Stage 4: Misadventure – characterised by a person choosing or being forced to participate in challenges beyond their capabilities resulting in negative emotions (fear, hurt, etc.), possibly injury or even death.[187]

As walk leaders, we manage risk: we manage the gap between real risk and perceived risk. We need to do that for every group and every individual on every occasion, with no assumptions. Every group is different, every venue is different and every person is different, so we really need to pay attention to so much. I cannot emphasise this enough: **we need to be fully present** and switched on ourselves. It is imperative that we know our forest very intimately, and we need skill and experience in assessing the situation carefully and predicting or anticipating needs. Our risk assessment is also dynamic and ongoing, so that we are alert to changes in any aspects or criteria that may impact the group. Both physical and emotional or psychological risk is meant in this context, and they have similar requirements in terms of our responsibilities and management practices.

There is a recent surge in counsellors and therapists being drawn to take therapy sessions outdoors without a sound understanding of the environment, or a deep familiarity with all its elements and vicissitudes. Partially because of this personal unfamiliarity, they may then have a tendency towards keeping everything really safe and limited and 'nice'. This may be presented or considered as a need to keep the client safe, contained, and within their comfort zone, but I challenge therapists to consider their own relationships with Nature and how much they are projecting their own fear. If we deprive our clients and participants of raw contact with Nature, then why are we out there in the first place? It could be that just leaving the relative comfort of the treatment room feels risky enough, but please check who is at risk and why, and what are the perceived threats or hazards versus the real dangers.

Efforts to make encounters with Nature safe or limited or 'nice', results in a very watered-down, anaesthetised version of the real thing, a simulacrum of Nature in its totality. We need to embrace risk, we need to encourage risk in our charges, and we need to be prepared like magicians to manage risk in a sleight-of-hand conjuring trick, where we know exactly where the edges are, and the client perceives a strong edge, but in reality is a long, safe distance from that edge. Sometimes that edge is physical: a path with a steep drop, a walk in the woods at night, taking a pee in the woods, climbing a tree. Sometimes the edge is more mental, emotional, and internal: stepping into the unknown, stepping beyond that ring fence of parental control into self, into what's forbidden or disapproved of.

If we are comfortable with our own relationship to risk, this feels like fertile territory for exploration, and we can relax into guiding others towards their wild edges, revealing the lost, abandoned, playful, and expansive outer skin of the animal. Imagine that a person has never walked barefoot in the woods, maybe not even as a child. You can hear the chiding parental voice saying, 'Don't get your clothes dirty, stay away from the mud.' And then one day, as an adult, they curiously turn up for a forest bathing session, and they are invited to take their shoes and socks off and go barefoot in the pine needles and the soil.

It's presented just as an invitation, it's not compulsory, but the person thinks, 'Here is an opportunity to do what was never allowed, I wonder what will happen? I hate the sight of my feet, I feel silly, how will I get clean and dry again? I can't be bothered, it's stupid and hippy, maybe I can just give it a go and at least say I've done it once. OK here goes, everyone else is relaxed about this nakedness of feet, they won't notice me.' And then there is that sublime almost erotic moment when the bare, unshod, starving foot first makes contact with the cool, soft welcoming soil, and the two embrace like long-lost lovers; a sensual shudder ripples up the spine, the feet talk to the brain, 20,000 sense receptors switch on, circuits light up, and the body says, 'Ahhhhhhh, I know that feeling', the hunter's feet reborn. This experience can serve as a strong catalyst for other acts of rebellion or exploring new aspects of life, or just become a little ritual the person chooses to continue themselves, removing the footwear whenever possible to feel that contact with earth – it's a form of liberation.

Embrace risk, understand risk, be prepared to allow risk, and take risk yourselves, it takes practice. I notice that we as a society are loathe to allow our children to take risks, but it really is our key role as parents to monitor the edge and manage the education of riskiness with our children, to encourage their curious expansive exploration of their new world. We teach them that fire burns, but it is also a magical, enchanting element. As they gain familiarity with fire from a very young age, they quickly absorb that learning into their subconscious: this is what I can do with fire, and this is what happens when I mess with fire. They then know the nature of fire, respect it, and value it as a part of themselves; fire is internalised. We don't seem to respect anything anymore because everything is dispensable, but Fire is a god, so why not show respect and welcome that energy appropriately into our hearts?

The same applies with sharp knives and tools: we teach children (and adults) what they are to be used for, how to use and not abuse them, and how to avoid cutting ourselves or each other. The same goes for cliffs, water, animals, and plants – we teach them respect for their physical world. Young brains are designed to rapidly take in this type of technical information and process it to form a picture of where those edges are, so that in later life, they already know the safe boundaries of risk, they intuitively trust their own judgements, and they can transfer those skills to other situations. Rather than trying to neurotically protect them from every conceivable scenario from birth, we can be demonstrating good risk management so that it becomes incorporated into the developing brain.

Finally, we need to encourage our mental health groups to take more risks in the woods, but again just to reiterate: the activity that one group finds challenging another will find easy and vice versa. The level of perceived risk or challenge needs to be commensurate with the abilities and energies of each group.

On one of my walks, I get the whole group to help each other scramble down a rocky bank with a drop into the river at the bottom. It looks dramatic, but it is quite safe, so long as they all assist each other down: communication, touch, support, body awareness or proprioception, trust, and laughter all play a part in a very simple task. They are also mostly barefoot at this point too.

The key thing is that prior to the sudden vertical scramble, everyone is walking along a path, perhaps on their own in silence, ruminating on various things, not that aware of each other, or awkward about starting conversation, or just spacing out on the scenery, then, suddenly, everything comes into very sharp focus. They are paying full attention, their breathing changes, muscles switch on, the Savage Self switches on: they are feeling the ground, going on all fours, sliding down on their bums, gripping the rocks, touching the soil, smelling the broken vegetation, being alive – embodied presence right there like an intoxicant.

In that place, there is no room for thoughts other than those of survival and purpose, no superfluous perambulations of the mind or paranoid delusions, just engagement with a physical survival task. Boundaries disintegrate, people hold each other's hands, or support their feet or carry their bags; helping each other, talking, sharing – tribal, ancient, powerful.

And when they all arrive safely at the bottom next to the river, you can see the difference in their faces, you can see those barriers of separation broken down, a feeling of exhilaration and relief: 'We made it!' Many people say how much easier they found it by being barefoot and gripping the earth and rocks.

There is another easier path to the river for those who want to play it safe, but I don't tell them that, because then they would split up and not be a tribe in that moment. The shared experience is vital for group cohesion and bonding, and generating support for the challenges ahead.

On my training courses, I emphasise the essential need to incorporate risk into the forest bathing walk. This is completely different to the more trad-itional way of walk leading in Japan, but my emphasis is different in terms of desired outcomes, cultural norms, and interpretation of Nature: always seeking the primitive, the feral play of the fox cubs and the instinctive self, and welcoming the edge of wildness back to our comfortable, polished lives.

In terms of personal risk, it feels essential that we reclaim the right to take risks in our lives, to not settle for the safe option each time. I'm not inferring the need for high-adrenaline cliff hanging (done that); it can be something as simple as taking off your socks and shoes, or allowing someone to lead you round with your eyes closed – it can be your version of perceived risk. It is the risk to be oneself, to be vulnerable in Nature.

The opposite of welcoming risk is numbness, we become the walking dead (we have become, as Pink Floyd sang 'comfortably numb'). When we swap the adventurous and unknown, therefore uncontrolled, element of our lives for comfort, we insulate ourselves from Nature, from wildness and life. People are absolutely fascinated by wild Nature, they will show up in their hoards to see some rare demonstration of wild Nature because it resonates deep within our forgotten switched-off feral cells and gives us hope of some freedom from the yoke of banality. 'As de Saussure said, risk-taking brings with it its own reward: it keeps a "continual agitation alive" in the heart. Hope, fear. Hope, fear.'[188]

We are hardwired for risk; our hunter-gatherer forebears knew that going out to search for food entailed risk at some level. If we turn our backs on risk and keep within our comfort zone, we forego all the strong, subtle qualities that made us successful, and we close down our horizons; we become small, compliant, weak, post-industrial herd animals. By adopting the philosophy of integrating risk into our lives, we wake up to who we are and we become mentally focused in the present. We accept that we might fail, appear foolish or embarrassed, but the rewards outweigh the negatives, because now we are firmly in touch with the inherited qualities and instincts we were born with.

Risk confronts apathy, risk opposes the slow banal death of suburbanised minds, risk that is informed from the intuitive guiding self leads to growth and self-knowledge. The play-it-safe pessimists of the world never accomplish much of anything, because they don't look clearly and objectively at situations, they don't recognise or believe in their own abilities to overcome even the smallest amount of risk.[189]

Recklessness is risk unmediated by the instinct, it is pure impulsiveness, or a deliberate overriding of those ancient survival mechanisms, and it too may serve some purpose, but that is not what I am advocating. Familiarity with risk enhances our ability to analyse and weigh up risk, and decide how to proceed. Trusting our instinctual Savage Self is about allowing the wise animal voice to guide us, so we can enjoy taking risks which enlarge and enhance our lives, and provide an antidote to the voices of fear, dread and mass paranoia that permeate our controlled lives and fearful attitudes.

Finally, and I know this may be slightly controversial, but consider that so long as it is very sudden, it is indeed a noble death to be killed by a tree; an organic death of two beings that stretch between Earth and heaven. A tragedy but a clean death.

I invite you to be fully present, to risk a little in life, risk showing up, being seen, being fully who you are; as Helen Keller wrote, 'life is either a daring adventure or nothing'. Please explore with sensual and creative freedom and less restraint, trust your inner instincts, and allow your senses to guide you, balance you, and enjoy this daring adventure and challenge of being truly alive. Enjoy the edges of the unknown.

CHAPTER 13

The Savage Self

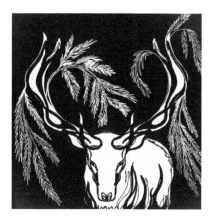

We are not just rather like animals; we are animals. Our difference from other species may be striking, but comparisons with them have always been, and must be, crucial to our view of ourselves.

MARY MIDGLEY[190]

I want to preface this section by acknowledging that I may offend at least a dozen different disciplines, including ethology, sociology, philosophy, and biology, not to mention individual sentiments, and will likely be shot down in flames for my lack of 'scientific proof' for this particular theory, but my hope is that by assembling a strong collection of somewhat disparate perspectives, the overlapping space in the middle of these will emerge to support the veracity of my claims. The truth of the existence of which is not essential for an acceptance of its overall purpose and value, namely to demonstrate that we are all still very much connected/hardwired to the various evolutionary phases that we have emerged from, and that our sense of distance and distinction from the rest of the biosphere is largely due to cultural myopia.

This chapter explores how we can perceive the benefits of forest bathing in relation to our innate animal survival response mechanisms. The focus of these mechanisms is to protect life, and prevent attack or predation by detecting, monitoring, and responding to threat. These mechanisms, although largely dormant, blunted, or unconscious, are nevertheless still a vital and demonstrative element of our evolutionary consciousness. I posit that we could not function fully without the support and learning from these primordial protectors.

We share a deep kinship with all of life, and whilst that connection may be relatively obvious in terms of our nearest cousins, the bonobos and chimpanzees, with whom we share 98.7 per cent of our DNA, is it possible that by digging a bit deeper we can discover more about our origins and the aetiology that links us to other forms of life that seem somehow very different from us? After all we *are*, as Mary Midgeley reminds us, animals, we are mammals, we are primates and we are bipedal monkeys; in spite of all our sophistications and extraordinary powers, we are still very much hardwired genetically as apes.

Biophilia applied

Biologists and neuroscientists predict survival optimisation responses based on complex interactions between the nervous system and regions of the brain including hardwired defence systems in the midbrain, alongside cognitive appraisal systems and vicarious learning. However, our more primitive fight, flight, or freeze responses come from phylogenetically older parts of the brain/nervous system. I propose that our primary platform for hierarchical responses to threat comes collectively from the gut-brain axis, including the enteric nervous system (ENS) and our genetically inherited instincts and intuition held within these evolutionary structures.

I term this innate mechanism the *Savage Self*. I hope to demonstrate in this chapter the importance of understanding our primal responses to fear and threat, and how being in the forest can create both biophilic and biophobic responses, and the relationship with chronic or non-specific anxiety states. After further description of the Savage Self, I will attempt to link this theme with a foundation of understanding our physiological and psychological relationship to Nature, as described in Stephen R. Kellert and E.O. Wilson's foundational book *The Biophilia Hypothesis*.[191]

The Savage Self is a term I have applied to a sense of inner or innate intelligence, a somatic knowing that derives from our repository of ancestral survival experiences going as far back as our mineral states, but most commonly associated with the evolutionary journey from primate to early hominid to Palaeolithic ancestor memories. Basically, what constitutes evolution, not adaptation.

The Savage Self has the capacity to shortcut the thinking, analytic, decision-making higher-functioning aspects of the brain when immediate direct threat is perceived and direct action is required in order to avoid danger. We can mobilise instantaneously when required and draw upon untapped reserves of strength in order to perform what would be considered superhuman tasks in everyday life, such as when a distraught mother lifts a car off her run-over child.

Unfortunately, this Savage Self has largely become a vestigial aspect of self, demoted in favour of a false sense of security; we trust rules and regulations and health and safety pronouncements, in the same way that we trust sat navs to tell us where we are going, and so lose the capacity to read maps or more basically orientate ourselves in space. We no longer fear the stalking sabre-toothed tiger, we don't look where we are going because we presume the pavement to be flat and without obstructions, and we no longer need to pay attention to all the vast sensory influx giving us rich, detailed three-dimensional information about our environment whilst we doodle on our phone.

Biophilia was a term used at the turn of the 20th century to refer to 'an instinct for self-preservation or the instinctual drive to stay alive'.[192] In the 1980s, Edward Wilson deployed the term to describe our innate affiliation with Nature and natural systems. Biophilia is important because it establishes an ethical and spiritual basis for the preservation of all life forms. Wilson argues that our innate attraction (*philia*) and tendency towards Nature is a biologically expressed need, which has become integral to our development and evolution as a species. Our strong responses and predispositions towards living things are part of our genetically conditioned survival mechanisms and have contributed towards the development of language through symbols and metaphors, culture, and our aesthetic value and appreciation of Nature, and therefore our healing and wellbeing (see Roger Ulrich's work on this).[193]

For the vast majority of our human evolutionary history, we have co-existed with Nature in small groups of hunter-gatherers; we looked and moved very differently to the *Homo sapiens* of today, we had a very finely tuned sense of our surroundings, and our survival depended on our instinctive and intimate knowledge of our environment, constantly updated through sensory inputs (see Chapter 10, The Senses).

We are still genetically hunter-gatherers and our bodies seek out optimal environments for food, water, and shelter. In a modern city, our Palaeolithic survival mechanisms read the city as an alien and hostile environment which causes us to go into chronic stress. In his wonderful book *Primate Change*, Vybarr Cregan-Reid examines the evolution of the hominid and the complex architecture of our bodies. He thinks that the way we are living and the adaptations we are making are not evolutionary. He comments:

> The overwhelming vast majority of our history has been spent hunter-gathering...the time since the Industrial Revolution...the time in which we have been doing sedentary work; we think of them in human terms and they seem normal...but they are such a small part of our history.
>
> As a result our bodies are in shock from these changes... Our bodies are defending and deforming themselves in response. Our limbic systems pump us full of nervous tension because they find themselves in urban environments they do not recognise. These environments seem normal to us at a conscious level, but on an unconscious one they lack traditional foraged sources of food and water, and so, as far as our primitive brains are concerned, they believe we have chosen to settle in a spartan desert.[194]

As we became settled agrarians, we brought all that accumulated nous with us and created myths and stories to remember our ancestral past and the monsters we faced. We began to forget our wild skills, our place within the community of beings; we were one step removed from our biological template, and we turned our learned survival strategies into warfare. We developed elaborate rituals to appease the new gods. Ultimately, we lost our tenuous conscious link to the past when we migrated to the cities as part of the Industrial Revolution, a process that is still happening in other parts of the world today. Yet Kellert and Wilson remind us: 'Biophilic rules persist from generation to generation, atrophied and fitfully manifested in the artificial new environments into which technology has catapulted humanity.'[195]

Another way of perceiving this shift in our purpose and adaptation or domestication process is through philosophy:

> Christianity taught us to see the eye of the Lord looking down upon us. Such forms of knowledge project an image of reality, at the expense of reality itself. They talk figures and icons and signs, but fail to perceive forces and flows. They bind us to other realities, and especially the reality of power as it subjugates us. Their function is to tame, and the result is the fabrication of docile and obedient subjects.[196]

From as early as I can remember, I have sensed this energy compelling me to go where I need to go, and do what I need to do, regardless of what I am being told, or told off for. I was strongly at odds with my Christian upbringing and have had to purge Catholicism from my system as an adult to remove guilt. I always had some very strong internal force directing me to follow where Nature leads, immersed in a dream state of bliss and curiosity, my inner guidance showing preferences towards particular habitats, creatures, plants, and trees, and away from others that didn't feel right.

This preternatural identification with Nature was heaven for little me until I went to school and then stood out like a sore thumb as being 'weird' and mostly socially incompetent. Luckily, that thread of rebellious undomesticated wildness has remained with me, and yet it often places me outside of what seems a strange and alluring society – a strong desire to belong running counter to my constant unrelenting peregrinations and unsubjugated urges. I somehow never acquired the capacity to be a 'docile and obedient subject'.

Ontogeny and phylogeny

The *Oxford Concise English Dictionary* defines savage as:

- adjective

  1. (of an animal or force of nature) fierce, violent, and uncontrolled: *packs of savage dogs roamed the streets*.

  2. *dated or offensive* (of a person or group) primitive and uncivilized: *a savage race*. (of a place) wild-looking and inhospitable; uncultivated.

- noun

  1. *dated or offensive* a member of a people regarded as primitive and uncivilized.

  2. *Heraldry* a representation of a bearded and semi-naked man with a wreath of leaves.

This dictionary definition makes me laugh with the images it conjures up of wild dogs, inhospitable tribes, and semi-naked bearded men roaming around; I say yes, let's have more of all that! The word's origin is from the Old French *sauvage* 'wild', via the Latin *silvaticus* 'of the woods', from *silva* 'a wood'.

As you can see from its etymology, 'savage' is a part of the wild: *sauvage*, part of the forest, *sylvanus* or *sylvaticus*, so I am reclaiming it as a positive aspect to embrace and explore. The dictionary puts a negative colonialist slant on this term because of the existential threat to the institution that the word poses, and the need to suppress or denigrate the word and the dark, mythic wild it represents.

It's worth remembering that Sylvanus is the tutelary god of the forest, he is the protective deity of the woods, and he particularly delights in trees growing wild. His ancient Greek counterpart is Pan, god of the wild places, meadows, sacred groves, wooded glens, and rustic music, and associated with fertility and the Spring (he is also seen as a sex god). The origin of the word Pan may go back to earlier Sanskrit texts meaning 'to protect, guard over', hence his affinity with shepherds. Sylvanus, Faunus, Pan are the gentle but fierce, savage embodiments of the Earth spirit living on in small enclaves of wilderness within increasingly complex civilisations.

Through this rendering, personification, and deifying of observed collective qualities of wild forces, we not only arrive at early belief systems but can understand more deeply the time before the 'great separation', a time when there was just forest, or when *Us* meant all of life together. 'Savage' then refers to the wild, untamed, and ancient protective energy of the Earth, inculcated within our DNA over thousands of generations of collective reverence and interdependence.

The Savage Self is the part of us that knows what to do: it's a primal, instinctive, incisive, vestigial aspect of our innate survival mechanism. It's the internal gyroscope that keeps us stable and alert, the part of us that has developed over many millions of years as a repository of all the accumulated evolutionary nous of our mineral, plant, animal, and hominid ancestors. It is both an abstract concept and a real visceral location within the centre of our body: 'Each person is at each moment capable of remembering all that has ever happened to him and of perceiving everything that is happening everywhere in the universe.'[197]

I have a gut feeling

This deep primal connection that exists between our brain and our gut is often referred to as the gut-brain axis or GBA. Our gut and brain have an extensive network of neurons connecting the central nervous system (CNS) with the enteric nervous system (ENS) which runs from the oesophagus to the anus. The GBA involves complex bidirectional communication between the cognitive and emotional centres in the brain (largely controlled by the limbic system), the endocrine and immune systems, and the activation of the sympathetic/parasympathetic nervous systems.

The concept that the gut and the brain are closely connected, and that this interaction plays an important part not only in gastrointestinal function but also in certain feeling states and in intuitive decision making, is deeply rooted in our language… From an evolutionary standpoint, it is clear that the enteric nervous system (ENS) is not uniquely human or even mammalian: homologues of an ENS are found throughout the animal kingdom, including in insects, snails and marine polyps.

It has been suggested that the ganglia that form the primitive brains of helminths, and eventually the brains of higher mammals, were derived from the more primitive but homologous enteric nerve circuits. Thus, neural circuitries and transmitter systems that have evolved to assure optimal responses (approach and withdrawal responses) to the challenges presented by our internal – for example, luminal – environment may have been incorporated into the CNS during evolution.[198]

Scientists are only just beginning to explore the mind-gut axis connection and realise how much our gut and microbiome influence our brain and our overall wellbeing. We have around two million neurons concentrated in the gut, about the equivalent of a dog's brain, and that is exactly the amount of intelligence we need down there to be a highly efficient mammal/primate/apex predator. There is no need for complex self-actualisation and philosophical contemplation when we have to act spontaneously and instinctively.

We often talk about having a 'gut feeling' or 'gut instinct': that's the Savage Self stepping in to inform us, alert us to potential threat, and take split-second evasive action when required without the head-brain intervening (which would involve weighing up all the options and take far too long). The Savage Self is situated in the middle of the body to cut down on synapse reaction times to each of the limbs. The Savage Self wasn't designed to help you write a poem or advise your dating choices, but it is designed to save your life in a threatening situation.

The enteric nervous system (ENS) is the third branch of the autonomic nervous system. It has the capacity to operate and 'think' independently of the CNS; it has about 500 million neurons, and bidirectional communication happens between the two via the vagus nerve pathway. People refer to the gut-brain as the second brain, but that is a hubristic misnomer, because in evolutionary terms the gut preceded the brain and evolved the gut-brain over millions of years. The ENS developed the CNS in order to control what was entering the gut via the mouth, hence the proximity of the two in most animals. The gut-brain also evolved in intimate mutual association with the microbiome of the gut: there are more microbes in our gut (estimated in the tens to hundreds of trillions) than there are stars in the Universe.

In some ways, you could say that the microbes are part of the environment, and gut flora cells vastly outnumber our human cells, so we are more environment than human, and not a separate entity to Nature. Our gut microflora and our gut-brain have happily evolved together in a mutually synergistic partnership over many millions of years, adapting to our changing environments, diets, and stressors. Maybe the gut microbiome has intelligence, and purpose.

Emerging evidence of the links between the microbiome and the CNS demonstrate how the ecosystem and composition of the gut microflora influences not only brain development, function, and behaviour, e.g., mood, but also mental health and a number of seemingly unrelated issues such as schizophrenia, type 2 diabetes, Parkinson's disease and autism.[199]

Conversely the emotions and moods of the individual can have an impact on overall gut health and microbiota balance. Chronic stress has been linked with intestinal permeability (leaky gut syndrome), which can in turn be linked to depression.[200] Diet and digestive system activity may affect cognition, and there is emerging evidence of how certain bacteria influence brain chemistry by secreting neuroactive compounds that have the capacity to affect sleep, appetite, metabolic function, and memory.[201]

The gut is also responsible for approximately 95 per cent of serotonin production, and serotonin affects mood, metabolism, muscle efficiency, and protein absorption. In summary, our gut microbiota play important roles in human physiology and pathology.

When I Was the Forest

When I was the stream, when I was the
forest, when I was still the field,
when I was every hoof, foot,
fin and wing, when I
was the sky
itself,
no one ever asked me did I have a purpose, no one ever
wondered was there anything I might need,
for there was nothing
I could not
love.
It was when I left all we once were that

the agony began, the fear and questions came,
and I wept, I wept. And tears
I had never known
before.
So I returned to the river, I returned to
the mountains. I asked for their hand in marriage again,
I begged – I begged to wed every object
and creature,
and when they accepted,
God was ever present in my arms.
And He did not say,
'Where have you
been?'
For then I knew my soul – every soul –
has always held
Him.

MEISTER ECKHART (1260–1328)

This wonderful poem by Meister Eckhart has an amazing contemporary quality to it, although written over 700 years ago. The poem alludes to this idea that we have been every part of the evolutionary process, and we too are intimately, phylogenetically comprised of all the different aspects of consciousness as they manifest in myriad phenomena or physical forms like sky, water, earth, trees, and animals (or 'beasts' as philosopher Mary Midgley calls them).

That is the whole point of life, surely, to recognise and revere our ancestors in terms of all planetary and evolutionary creative expressions. They are quite literally our parents, stars are our parents, and we have become childish, rather than child-like, full of entitlement, rather than innocence and awe. But the fundamental energy of the Universe is unconditional love, so we are deeply cared for, even in our rejection of life and our technological cynicism, and as we express our wills to their limits.

As early hominids, we had relatively few resources to protect ourselves from attack from other predators. We possess neither big sharp claws nor teeth, strong jaws, strong legs, or the ability to run fast. It's true our ancestors were much stronger than us and had much larger jaws, but even so, we were no match for the sabre-toothed tiger or an angry mammoth. What about another tribe wanting to eat us? We could climb once, but for how long could we remain arboreal without coming to the ground?

What we do have is this instinctive aspect which is constructed from the repository of stored ancient knowledge deep within the DNA of our being. Our instincts and intuition are composite survival memories across multi-species ancestry. These instinctive responses were our supreme sensory superpower and what alerted us to immediate or impending threat, when we were listening to that subtle voice. Other creatures have similar methods of prey detection, or predator awareness – you often hear this referred to as them sensing when 'something isn't quite right.' (My poor dog seemed to know a few hours before it was his bath time and would run away.)

We still have all those atrophied faculties, and occasionally they are able to break through into consciousness to warn or alert us to something, an alarm to pay attention or to not follow a particular path. If we hadn't felt with them, we wouldn't be here still. It was a very long time before we developed weapons and fire to defend and hunt more effectively; we relied on our keen senses and intuition. We could sense the vibrations on the ground and in the air if threat was near. If the birds went quiet, we understood it was time to run or fight.

Midgley argues that before the invention of tools and weapons, we would have found it difficult to kill another human successfully in the way that a carnivore like a wolf or lion could dispatch another animal. Therefore, we did not develop the inhibitions or restraints shown by other top predators towards aggressive acts. Once we had weapons, it was too late to develop moral boundaries for our behaviours; ironically, we refer to our less than caring behaviours as 'beastly', 'bestial', 'savage', or 'animal'. In fact, there are relatively few examples from the animal kingdom of random unprovoked attacks or uncontrolled aggression.

Most animals know that it is far better to run away and avoid confrontation, or to establish a clear hierarchy of power; males may battle to the death for mating rights but be otherwise fairly placid. Animals have natural evolutionary laws which govern their behaviour, but historically our mono-theistic religion and the influence of Cartesian duality has taught us that we are the superior species on the planet, and that the beasts and plants were put there for our edification and consumption.[202]

We fear and mythologise many animals, particularly those that would eat us, whilst failing to see that we too have been largely responsible for the wholesale slaughter of animals, beyond our immediate perceived needs for food. We routinely and randomly kill en masse, because we have distanced ourselves from the souls and the nobility of these creatures, and our fellow humans, and from any sense of our belonging in the pantheon of beasts. And yet we have also not acquitted ourselves well when considering our position regarding our presumed superiority and custodianship of the flora and fauna of the biosphere: our innate humanity that elevates us from the 'savages' is an abstract concept, not real.

We use the term 'savage' to indicate a person without morality or religion, a person outside of society and therefore lacking in rules, manners, and reason. Primitive and uncivilised, as the dictionary tells us, but when we interrogate that assumption we find the truth to be different. Since the time when we set off in search of far-distant lands to conquer, we have encountered other iterations of the human species, tribes and cultures alien to our own. Some of those encounters have gone well, and some, possibly most, have ended in bloodshed or the transfer of diseases to indigenous peoples who had no resistance or immunity to them. We regarded these other peoples as savages because their lifestyles, cultures, and beliefs were so different from ours, we decimated or enslaved them, and they did their own share of internecine warfare too. Let's not mythologise the savage but see within these early tribal cultures the seeds of our own morality.

Midgley argues that the way we demonise the beast without is commensurate with the way we demonise the beast within.[203] To me, these are simply projections of shadow aspects, the unintegrated parts of our own evolutionary impulses that allow us to distance ourselves from these base instincts, scapegoat the beast within, and align ourselves with a virtuous God, and a justifiable cause. Midgley suggests primitive man had weak inhibitions, would perhaps kill others and then feel remorse for his actions, and that thinking about ways to avoid conflict arose as the precursors to intelligent social reasoning and rules of morality.

In the wild, dominant wolves show restraint when the conquered enemy demonstrates the body language of submission, which is often a mimicking of a very young animal's behaviour. I would therefore suggest that we too must have some degree of impulse restraint that has been suppressed or discounted in our martial narratives. The larger point here is that the term 'savage' has been misinterpreted as a pejorative abstract based on fundamental misrepresentations of animals and other tribes in order to hypocritically distance ourselves from the very behaviours that we alone are indiscriminately capable of.

When we are not generally exposed to a real immediate threat (which is probably most of us right now), we tend to switch off or tone down our outer and inner senses; we relax, abdicate responsibility for our safety to the great Health and Safety god and his regulations, and assume a cohesive level of socially acceptable freedom from harm and threat. These protective policies and fundamental principles are an important aspect of urbanised conditioning, but the assumptions they promulgate lead us into a false sense of protection and security, because things can always go wrong (see Chapter 12, Risk).

Since we no longer have our sensibilities switched on, our primitive radars of threat have been blunted, rendered redundant, and with them our innate wisdom and comprehension of the world we are part of – the world of spirit and matter, the world of the unconscious (the community of the wild soul), and its common mutual language of symbols with Nature. By replacing superstition with logic and science, we have in our sophistication lost our path and our core; our strong, listening, sensuous Savage Self has gone into deep hibernation. This vestigial and protective power remains dormant, on standby, until we face a sudden threat.

As we begin to spend more time out in Nature, that archaic voice awakens from its slumbers, becomes aware of its functioning ecological environment; the Savage Self begins to stir in response to the wilder stimuli and familiar elemental landscapes of pre-industrial consciousness. The Savage Self is so much more than just a visceral response or extension of our limbic systems, rather, it's better to consider that the limbic system is in service of the Savage Self. The limbic system (limbic means edge or border, and has the same root as liminal – threshold) first appeared about 150 million years ago and marks an evolutionary transformation from the reptilian brain to the more advanced mammalian brain.

The limbic system's development went hand in hand with new evolutionary modes of being and social interaction. It is an extension of the ENS, a sort of external hard drive for the gut-brain, which propelled refinement from reptilian to more complex mammalian ways of being in the world. The limbic system matches memories and behaviours from past experiences with present events, however, most of the information held by the parts of the limbic system is innate, not learned. We are born with it; it is ancestral.

These innate behaviours are linked to emotions and include mating, maternal instincts, defence against predators and the establishment of social hierarchies, all of which ensure survival of the individual, or offspring and propagation of the species.[204] This innate template of knowledge that we are born with is what fascinated the early philosophers, such as Thales (see Chapter 3).

The limbic system, intuition, and ENS (collectively the Savage Self) rely on external senses (of which smell may have been the most critical; see Chapter 10) and internal senses such as proprioception, to modify behaviours according to perception and stimulus, building a three-dimensional synaesthetic picture of the environment. I think one of the reasons why *shinrin-yoku* practices improve wellbeing outcomes is due to this deep ancient connection being reactivated through sensory stimulation.

The instinctive or intuitive (non-linear) decision-making draws on the rich library of vestigial survival experiences in the ancestral memories held within this primal core. Ernst Haeckel's now-defunct and disproved theory 'ontogeny recapitulates phylogeny', which posited that developing human embryos experience many of the different evolutionary transitions of the animal kingdom, starting as a small single cell, growing into a zygote and then moving through the major phyla, or taxonomical groups, does have a thread of truth in it, as scientists have revealed that developing babies in the womb have extra lizard-like muscles in their hands and feet that most will lose before they are born. They are probably one of the oldest, albeit fleeting, remnants of evolution seen in humans yet, biologists say in the journal *Development*.[205] They date them as 250 million years old, a relic from when reptiles transitioned to mammals.

It is thought that we may have around one hundred such vestigial memories expressed in different ways, and many are lost before or after birth. Examples include:

- the Moro or startle reflex in babies

- the tails that embryos grow at about six weeks

- our wisdom teeth which are remnants of when we had larger jaws and a third set of molars

- the additional muscles that some people have in their arms which are thought to be used for gripping and hanging.

Intuition

Intuition is neither a feeling, an inspiration nor a disorderly sympathy but a fully developed method.

GILLES DELEUZE[206]

Intuition is described as the ability to acquire knowledge without recourse to conscious reasoning. Different fields use the word intuition in very different ways, such as direct access to unconscious knowledge, unconscious cognition, inner sensing, inner insight to unconscious pattern recognition, and the ability to understand something instinctively, without any need for conscious reasoning.[207]

The word intuition comes from the Latin *intueri* meaning 'to consider', but if you can allow me this whimsical idea, I like to think intuition can be split into *inner* and *tuition* – *inner-tuition*. This means that we have this ability to learn from what lies deep inside us beneath our conscious control, a reservoir of largely untapped wisdom from our ancestral past. Jung was also curious about this aspect of our psyche. He describes intuition as a sense-perception and a 'hunch', an involuntary event dictated by external or internal circumstances. He describes intuition as being irrational, not in a negative sense, but to differentiate it from the rational, i.e., thinking and ordering acts as opposed to perceiving acts: 'it depends essentially upon objective stimuli, which owe their existence to physical and not to mental acts.'[208]

Intuition is a kind of super-perception or extrasensory perception that can read energies and objective stimuli, and communicate at a subconscious level with the rest of the body, distinct from the ego-self. The smartest way to avoid life-threatening encounters is to detect them before they can happen and then take evasive action. Nowadays that can translate into not taking that flight, not setting off on that journey, not going back to that person's house, a hunch to go and visit a friend or family member, and so on.

The best form of martial art is to defeat your enemy before they get to within a hundred miles of you, before they have even thought to attack you. Our ancestors learned to attune to trouble using this wonderful psychic radar, an apparatus evolved through natural selection and strongly present in some people more than others (the 'seers').

Intuition is nothing but a fleeting glimpse or sensation without that relationship with the instincts of the body, and the capacity to mobilise our resources in a split second if our radar detects imminent threat. If you think about this colossal and 'haphazard' evolutionary journey that we have been on since the Big Bang, and that somehow we are one of the most advanced technologies to exist in the Universe (that we know of), it makes sense that we would also have developed some fairly sophisticated defence mechanisms – we are indeed precious evolutionary cargo.

This protective survival mechanism is our source of power, and it is our connection to both human and non-human kinfolk, our membership of the collective and imaginal realms. All life came from one common point of origin; we are all linked, we are all on a path together. Our egos like to trick us into believing in our separation and individualism, but the collective unconscious is the repository of our communal experiences and stories as expressed by the common archetypes shared by all cultures and societies.

At night, we dream together, and our dreaming rejoins us back to Nature, back to our intuition. In our 'night-consciousness', our wild god primeval self is unshackled from conscription and servitude. At night,

> we are confronted with an intuition of emotive origin, and we enter the nocturnal empire of a primaeval activity of the intellect which, far beyond concepts and logic, exercises itself in vital connection with imagination and emotion. We have quit logical reason and even conceptual reason. Yet we have to do more than ever with intuitive reason functioning in a non-rational way.[209]

The Savage Self is the black box recorder of each life handed down from one generation to another, and in our dreams we attempt to find psychic resolution for past events and ancestral traumas, alongside inspired imagination. Jung referred to dreams as 'pure nature', and we now know that the dreaming function in mammals is about 140 million years old and has a survival function[210] (see Human Givens in the section on 'The health benefits of *shinrin-yoku*', Chapter 7).

Jung writes:

> You are a collection of ancestral spirits, and the psychological problem is how to find yourself in a crowd... A human life is nothing in itself; it is part of a family tree. We are continuously living the ancestral life, reaching back for centuries, we are satisfying the appetites of unknown ancestors, nursing instincts which we think are our own, but which are quite incompatible with our character; we are not living our own lives, we are paying the debts of our forefathers... We go on as a historical compensation for ancestors... though we think they have nothing to do with our lives.[211]

Jung felt that instinct is a part of Nature and seeks to perpetuate Nature. He also believed that we are the carriers of the entire history of mankind.[212] I feel that we are the carriers of the entire history of the Universe, and given the gravity of that statement, it's strange that we choose to occupy ourselves with watching videos of cats jumping on sofas, whilst the planet slides towards disequilibrium and extinction for many species, us included. Jung realised how out of balance we had become one hundred years ago, and I think he would be shocked to witness what we have become today, but his compassionate analysis of modern man reveals how we are dissociated from Nature, and in need of healing.[213]

Jung refers to an Archaic man as our primitive antecedent, a being who lives much closer to our phylogenetic instinct,[212] a being more in tune with the cycle of the seasons, more likely to follow nature rather than go against it, both internally and externally. This ancient connection is reawakened when we have contact with the soil. We fall back into 'irrational', unconscious states that allow us to 'see' with animal eyes. Our intuitive capacities allow us to see beyond the normal perceptual range, while a powerful, largely unconscious feeling will place great value upon intuitive experience and not let it slip.[214]

Jung felt that the modern mind was concerned with causality, rationalism, and the hyper-masculine qualities associated with a linear, left-brained approach to life, with Nature distrusted, it representing the chaotic, dark, undifferentiated power of the feminine. I have experienced this myself so many times it cannot just be my misperception of a few vandalistic acts. They have manifested as a highly justified need to clean things up, make them accessible, presentable, tidy, conformist. I see their faces, I hear their logical justifications; it's all about safety, about stopping people getting lost. I see how affronted they are by this possibility of a slide into a feral cacophony of briars and burrs. I wrote a whole poem about this once.

The first time I became fully conscious of how it impacted me viscerally was when I was at Agricultural College doing my Environmental Education diploma. Across the lane from my college digs, there was a playing field, and beyond that an area of unvisited and abandoned woodland on the very boundaries of the college estate. Of course, it drew me in immediately and once inside I felt I had entered another world. The entrance was of particular interest because of its magical portal qualities. The whole front side that bordered the playing field was dense with brambles and impenetrable scrub. In the middle of that green boundary, there was a willow tree that had fallen over, but was still growing. Its two main trunks formed a perfect elliptical eye shape with darkness beyond, so that you would have to climb over one and under the other to gain entry to the woods: the eye of the woods, a perfect threshold of power.

Then one day one of my tutors, who was very cut off from his feeling self, very academic and science-focused, decided that with the forthcoming visit of some dignitary to the college, we should clear this area up. The whole protective green wall was cut down, exposing the delicate underbelly of the woods. It felt so violent – a transgression. It was devastating.

This attitude has been directed at the sacred sites in Cornwall. Some charity has taken it upon themselves to clear up all these sacred sites and signpost them. It's an utter disaster, and I feel the pain of these sensitive, feminine sites and how the briars, brambles and blackthorn thickets are there to protect and contain the energies and mysteries of these holy places. You are not meant to be signposted to these sites down a clearly defined track; you are meant to stumble upon them whilst lost, after hearing a whispered incantation calling across the fields, and struggling with all the thorns and prickles, so that when you arrive, you are suitably chastened and humble.

But man can't leave well alone and seeks to interfere at any opportunity due to this habitual modern fear of the unknown in Nature, this need to tidy everything up and make it neat, conditioning overriding instinct. Of course, 'as above, so below', and how we treat Nature and remain separate has been regarded by ecopsychologists as representative of how we respond to all those wild, unacknowledged parts of the feral and forest inside us. Where are our own internal sacred places and quiet hidden groves?

So, when we come to the forest and experience the immersive properties of *shinrin-yoku*, what has become evident to me over a 30-year period of guiding people therapeutically in Nature is that the deep, consciously intentional absorption in Nature eventually awakens the dormant voice of the Savage Self. Because it is us, it is the very essence of what drives us. When it's not required for survival, it is available as an internal gyroscope, bringing us back to our primal visceral sense of who we are. As I warn my students, this is not all love and light.

Becoming more in touch with this inner wild woman or man leads us away from neuroses, anxieties, and preoccupations that keep us tamed; we become paradoxically more compassionate towards others and also less tolerant of bullshit, of the excesses of a civilisation in decline. We become a lot fiercer, and that is a good thing. We may become perceived as a threat, as Jung recognised how this quality accrued through Nature connection and sensed how his closeness to Nature affected others:

> It is the truth, a force of nature that expresses itself through me – I am only a channel – I can imagine in many instances where I would become sinister to you.
>
> For instance, if life had led you to take up an artificial attitude, then you wouldn't be able to stand me, because I am a natural being. By my very presence I crystallize; I am a ferment. The unconscious of people who live in an artificial manner senses me as a danger. Everything about me irritates them, my way of speaking, my way of laughing.

They sense nature.[215]

I love this quote and Jung's use of the word *ferment*, defined as passion, anger, to boil and seethe.

George Monbiot also relates to this experience of shedding civilisation when he encounters a dead deer whilst out foraging. He realises a sudden connection to the sense of a genetic memory of hunting deer:

> while we were still subject to natural selection, we were shaped by impera-
> tives – the need to feed, defend and shelter ourselves, to reciprocate and
> work together, to breed and care for our children – which ensured that
> certain suites of behaviour became instinctive...they evolved to guide us.
> These genetic memories – these unconsidered urges – are printed onto our
> chromosomes, an irreducible component of our identity.[216]

Monbiot infers that the fierce aspect of the Savage Self and the instincts that once helped us to defend ourselves and our families from both preda-tors and competing clans are disastrous in a densely populated society. He considers the need 'to press our roaring blood into quieter channels'.[215] But this constriction is a major contributing factor to our malaise: 'where these urges are familiar to us, experience has taught us how to suppress or redirect them.' My invitation in the forest is to listen in to these urges, and be open and receptive to what they might reveal about our authentic nature, our wild truth, or, as Monbiot experienced it, 'overwhelming, raw, feral. I did not have a place to put it; but I knew that it belonged to me.'[215]

It belongs to all of us, we have all become enslaved by the sweet filed-down edges of domesticated complicity in this silent desperation. These untamed landscapes soon remind our bodies how it feels to be strong again, whole again. Intuition has been relegated to choosing bingo numbers, but it is our gift from before, our reconciliation to Spirit:

> The deeper gift of the fiery intuiter is the body itself, direct sense-perception
> that brings the high-flying spirit back to the present, the here-and-now; to
> the grounding, slow and deepening motions of the soul, to give life body and
> substance.[217]

How many of us can say that we are truly grounded day to day? We are skewed off centre by our over-stimulating environments; when we get to the woods, the slow, silent green and the slow-moving trees soothe the frantic psyche, and we come into rest and reflection. It is also here that we come into contact with the wilder archetypes of our inner savage.

This shift in momentum back to the genetically programmed pace allows the 'gift' to be revealed, a slowing down, a grounding, a squatting on the earth, the smell of soil getting stronger, intoxicating. We feel a dance, an involuntary movement from deep in the belly, that smooth muscle, that fierceness, the place of self-awareness, and the darker recesses of the personality come to the fore, our quorum sensing of inherited wealth and wise-dom.

Sit still or move from the body from the centre and the Savage Self is reactivated, it becomes an ally in your daily life, 'a transpersonal eco-Alexa'. We instinctively know (once we overcome our cultural fears) that we belong in the forest, that we are an intrinsic part of the ecosystem. When we step over that threshold into the woods, we step back in time and we step from a very mind and vision-dominated society into a world where our body has greater dominion over our lives, where Nature has greater dominion over our bodies, and where all of our senses are primed for an electric exchange. What gifts do you have to share with the forest?

The unbounded joyous freedom when the body-mind takes over, whether we are sitting, running, crawling in the leaves, or climbing the trees; we fall back into our evolutionary history, because as sophisticated as our contemporary lives are, our bodies are still part of another earlier epoch. Our animal selves shoehorned into numbing modernity are suddenly unleashed into a sensuously dynamic, glistening, kaleidoscopic environment that is mirrored in our cellular memory.

Wilhelm Reich believed that trauma, painful experiences and repressed or forbidden feelings, particularly around sexuality, were held in the muscles of the body and formed a layer of defensive 'armouring' which hardened our bodies over time, and showed up in our posture and movement. Reich's view was that neuroses and anxiety were held in the body, and so therefore, through working with the body directly, could be released. Over time, if not attended to, these patterns of holding develop into personality patterns and psychosomatic illnesses.

Reich observed that people do not surrender to the animal self, to an instinctual, involuntary urge of the body, partly through a fear of the unknown, or anxiety about the liberation of orgasm, thereby denying our bodies their full uninhibited expressions. Spending time in the forest invites us to let the body off the leash, to play, to become somatically present, to be sensuous. This coming into the body is a subversive act, being in Nature is an act of anarchy against the system which encourages us to dissociate from our bodies, and to discriminate against others based on their body shape, skin colour, and sexual orientation.

For Reich, true liberation can occur when we overthrow these oppressive patriarchal values that seek to commodify the body, and enjoy the right to free expression of our sexuality. This is a parallel process to that of deep engagement with Nature; we come into the body, we listen to the wise, pre-industrial voices of our ancestral and savage selves, and we experience a kind of orgasm of unity with all life. Being in Nature when we are in tune and uninhibited is a sexual experience, ergo a creative expression of Divine Intelligence.

The Savage Self may be hypothetical, but it is also a very real visceral gut location, a real, though not visible organ. It is the omphalos, the solar plexus, the confluence of both branches of the vagus nerve, the third or Manipura chakra from the Vedic traditions of India, and is regarded as connected to our sense of self, sense of purpose, and identity.

It is the billions-of-years-old collaboration between our spirits and the stars, the millions-of-years-old collaboration between our nervous system and the trillions of microbes within our internal microbiome. Ultimately, it is a primary, united, undifferentiated voice of Nature, a forest tongue speaking from within us, neglected, yet available for our inner guidance, wellbeing and survival.

I will leave the last word to that stalwart of the environmental movement and one of my first heroes, Rachel Carson:

> As human beings, we are part of the whole stream of life. We have been human beings for perhaps a million years. But life itself passes on something of itself to other life – that mysterious entity that moves and is aware of itself and its surroundings, and so is distinguished from rocks or senseless clay – [from which] life arose many hundreds of millions of years ago. Since then it has developed, struggled, adapted itself to its surroundings, evolved an infinite number of forms. But its living protoplasm is built of the same elements as air, water, and rock. To these the mysterious spark of life was added. Our origins are of the earth. And so there is in us a deeply seated response to the natural universe, which is part of our humanity.[218]

CHAPTER 14

Lost

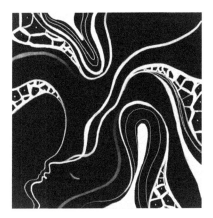

When you lose your path, a surge of excitement comes to both your mind and body; your calm shores begin to be beaten by the waves! This vitality created by being lost is a good incentive to get lost!

MEHMET MURAT ILDAN[219]

It is an important part of our ancient heritage and psychological development that we can allow ourselves the wonderful gift of getting lost from time to time. Before you all raise your arms in horror, let me qualify that by stating that getting lost in some countries can have disastrous consequences, and getting lost on the mountains, particularly in winter, can be fatal if you are unprepared. Getting lost in the woods of the UK poses very little risk, as if you just walk off in any direction, sooner or later you will encounter a road or a retail coffee outlet. In the US and other places with extensive wilderness, the ramifications of getting lost have to be fully understood before undertaking such a crazy venture.

Before we discuss practicalities, let's have a look at principles. Knowing where we are at all times has been drummed into us from an early age. If we occasionally make a wrong turn on the motorway, we fear never finding our way back home again. In recent years, there has been a growing reliance on sat nav and GPS tracking systems on our phones, and this dependence means that our natural navigator skills become ever more atrophied and lost.

We never really allow ourselves the chance to be fully lost physically, and so conversely we can never be truly found. I can remember an occasion when I was driving back across a city in the dark after dropping my daughter off, and I took a wrong turn. I didn't know where I was, or which street I was in, and in the dark I couldn't read my street map, so I did experience this visceral feeling of panic just for a moment before my senses kicked in and I then calmed down, trusted my wild navigation skills, and found my way back. So there is quite a distinction between being urban lost, which is qualitatively different, and *planned* Nature lost.

So, before we go any further, please switch the mobile phone off and bury it in the bottom of your daypack.

Being completely lost in Nature can be such a joy, and such an adventure when we are in the right frame of mind. The feeling of being lost is an important learning tool in Nature. First, we are suddenly liberated from all agendas and route directions and linear narratives, set free to wander and roam in any direction. Second, we are now supercharging all those semi-dormant senses; we are getting in the hunter's zone, ears pricked, skin tingling, eyes attuning to the subtleties and features of the topography. As hunters, we can move with meticulous economy; we begin to access ancient instincts for feeling where we are relative to the Earth's position, to north, to the running streams and the wind, the flight of the birds, and the inner sense of navigation.

When we follow the old familiar path, we close down our awareness of our ancient instinctual faculties, and our exposure to the exhilaration of the new, the unforeseen. The tender and unexplored parts of the earth-body reveal different smells, different songs, new vistas, new perspectives, and we are in the edge zone of our wild knowing and reciprocating with the gifts of this unexplored terrain. It's uncanny how the outer and inner landscapes can mirror each other, as if the skin were that permeable membrane of psychic exchange. The well-worn path gives us the safety of the habitual journey getting lost by contrast awakens our longing for the stimulation of the unknown.

Which way is the wind blowing? Where is the sun now? What are the animals around me doing? They're not lost; maybe I can go home with them? That first sensation of boundaryless liberation can feel daunting or ecstatic depending on your current temperament, but then something happens. You drop down into a state of connected personal authority, into the belly, into trust, you don't panic, you just breathe and set off on an adventure, albeit an adventure that might see you needing to clamber over walls, through bracken and briars, do some U-turns, cross streams and ditches, and generally get messy. This process is exceptionally good as an antidote to depression, especially if you can have a few rants and shake your fists at life whilst wading through a bog or stream.

Until you've experienced the sheer joy this brings, you are probably thinking that I'm completely irresponsible and that this description is bringing up terror and dread, but I urge you to give it a try. I fully understand that lone females may be apprehensive to do this, so you could have someone you know and trust to walk some distance off but keep you in their sights, or initially go with a friend who is happy to walk in silence with you.

Here's how to make it successful: start small and containable. In mountaineering navigation, we talk about 'hand rails'. A hand rail is a linear feature in the landscape that delineates a given area of land, e.g., fences, walls, rivers, roads, railway lines, ridges, or power lines. If we know roughly where these hand rails are, they give us a sense of containment within a given boundary. We just need three or four of them, and then we have an area to play with.

Have a look at the map – a physical map – preferably at a 1:25000 scale. Choose an area that you don't know at all, and then work out some macro features that will give that containment: there's a big wooded hill to the north, there's a small village to the south, an old canal in the east, and I'm setting off from the west. This area could be walked in just a couple of hours or keep you amused all day – you decide. Build up your confidence to just walk along without any sense of where you are going, what the time is, or where you will end up.

The point of all this cannot be easily explained here – you just have to do it, and see what happens. It creates a sort of magic that puts you in touch with the fully alive sensory palpations of your undulating ground. We are now wandering without purpose or direction, simply following our inner calling and our feral nose reading the scent of the trail. We are no longer just hiking through.

This reminds me of a famous John Muir quote about hiking:

I don't like either the word [hike] or the thing. People ought to saunter in the mountains – not 'hike'! Do you know the origin of that word saunter? It's a beautiful word. Away back in the Middle Ages people used to go on pilgrimages to the Holy Land, and when people in the villages through which they passed asked where they were going they would reply, 'A la sainte terre', 'To the Holy Land'. And so they became known as sainte-terre-ers or saunterers. Now these mountains are our Holy Land, and we ought to saunter through them reverently, not 'hike' through them.[220]

As we gain confidence, we can begin to saunter further afield; sometimes it's good to use a map, sometimes it's good to use a compass, sometimes it's good to just set off without anything except the sun, the moon, and the stars, and discover new parts of Nature (which of course, reveal new parts of ourselves). This discipline teaches us more about our own internal resources, our internal compass, our hidden strengths and determination, mixed with lightness and a no-agenda reality. It's a fluid way of being, it's feminine, it's challenging us to have faith. We are always in hiking mode in life, carrying a big pack, eyes to the ground, one foot in front of the other, so here's a chance to go differently.

Make sure you are prepared kit-wise – I can't stress this strongly enough. It's not responsible to set off without having the right kit with you, so as a minimum I recommend to take water, a waterproof, a warm sweater, a bite to eat and a spare snack bar. Other options include a head torch, whistle, hat, suncream, and notebook.

Gradually, build up your getting lost muscles and you will find it empowers you in other areas of your life. 'Staying alive in the woods is a matter of calming down.'[221] Getting lost in the forest is great because we have limited visibility, so actually a small area can be a great adventure, and we come to notice so much more, because we need to. This is an aspect of forest bathing you will not find in any literature about the subject, but this aimless meandering brings an added dimension to our practice.

Getting lost with a group also has its own challenges, especially if it wasn't intentional! However, deploying the 'Help, I'm lost' tactic can have very beneficial results for the bonding of the group, but only – and I stress only – after the group have been meeting for quite a period of time and have developed a strong relationship with you as leader and with each other. There needs to be a camaraderie between all of you first.

Go to a new area of woodland, and wander into the middle of the woods; they probably won't pay attention to where you are, or how you got there, especially if you went round in a circle. Stop the group and declare that you are lost and need their help to find your way to a place, or the way out. This gives them the chance to feel fully empowered as a group and for them to take responsibility; they are no longer passengers but drivers, coming together to sort it out.

Your ego might take a hit, but it is worth it to witness the change in dynamic and the communications that take place, who suddenly takes charge, who has the best plan, and who doesn't really care anyway. Of course, you won't be fully lost because you have your hand rails in place as boundaries, but you are facilitating the perception of being lost.

Finally, here is another perspective on getting lost, from a prayer of the First Nation tribes of North America, translated into a poem by American poet David Wagoner.

> Stand still. The trees ahead and bushes beside you
> Are not lost. Wherever you are is called Here,
> And you must treat it as a powerful stranger,
> Must ask permission to know it and be known.
> The forest breathes. Listen. It answers,
> I have made this place around you.
> If you leave it, you may come back again, saying Here.
> No two trees are the same to Raven.
> No two branches are the same to Wren.
> If what a tree or a bush does is lost on you,
> You are surely lost. Stand still. The forest knows
> Where you are. You must let it find you.[222]

CHAPTER 15

Conclusions

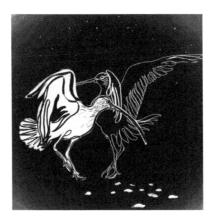

The Kogi people of what is now modern-day Colombia are a highly evolved tribe with incredible abilities. For centuries, from the top of their sacred mountain in Sierra Nevada de Santa Marta, they have felt the energy lines that are stretched out all across the Earth. Whenever they sense a small imbalance in Earth's energies, they attempt a rebalance by placing gold objects beneath the surface of the ground, almost like a large acupuncture pin, to restore harmony to the Earth.

When the Spanish conquistadors arrived, the peaceful, humble Kogi came to the beach to greet them. The explorers declared the land theirs in the name of the king of Spain, took away all the gold, and set their man-eating dogs free to attack the Kogi. The white man had arrived in the Americas.

Those that survived took refuge near the top of the mountain, and that is where they have largely stayed to this day, protected from visitors and intrusions from the outside world. They call us 'younger brother' and they are 'convinced that our ignorance and greed will destroy the balance of life on Earth'.[223]

They initially spoke to the world in the 1980s: they decided that they had witnessed and detected such devastation from their mountain that they wanted to send a message imploring us to change track and restore the balance to the Earth. They created two documentaries with Alan Ereira to help spread their message around the world. Their message is simple:

> They see the world as a single living being which they have to look after and care for. Their whole way of life is dedicated to nurturing the flora and fauna of the world; they are, in short, an ecological community whose morality is wholly concerned with the health of the Planet... The world is beginning to die. They know we are killing it.[222]

In the intervening 40+ years things have got worse – we are still not listening!

The ice caps are melting, smog blankets the whole planet, the sea is teeming with microplastics, humans are full of forever chemicals, and our fertility rates are plummeting, and every day the sanctity of the living Earth is violated a million times as we burn, bulldoze and poison our lands and forests, the lungs of the planet. Animals are going extinct at increasing rates.

This self-destructive behaviour has been likened to a form of madness caused by deep psychological trauma. Thelemists regard our behaviour as being that of a child god, spoiled, impetuous, entitled, and lacking self-awareness. Whatever the cause, we are not able to act wisely because we have become distanced from the kinds of feelings, behaviours, and values that are aligned with Nature. Over many generations, we have been adapted for purpose, anaesthetised, and desensitised to become dispensable tools in the profit machine.

We have long-term cultural amnesia, losing track of the animal and forager deep inside us; we have been engineered towards demonising and distancing ourselves from our true feral natures, employing elaborate dogmas, deceptions, doctrines, and rituals to keep us locked into the dream of becoming happy 'one day', whilst being deliberately alienated from our home on this Earth, and from practices of reverence towards the immediate, practical, and benevolent gods of the forest. The plant and animal spirits have been replaced by the two false gods of religion and science, who persistently fail to deliver on the end of suffering and the equality of all beings.

We can no longer hide and feign ignorance as the reminders of our folly are all around us, and the tools for choosing a new and wise, healthy path are also before us. We as individuals now have this responsibility, as our governments consistently fail to meet their promises on climate change and numerous other policies of social responsibility and commitments to low-impact energy systems. It has become incumbent on us to use our voice, and to speak up for Nature, to create change, to take brave, bold decisions for our planet and for our children. We will need to sacrifice consumption for joy, titillation for beauty, and arrogance and insularity for muck and mud – what's not to like?

Forest bathing and forest medicine present us with a relatively new and exciting opportunity to expand consciousness, develop pro-environmental behaviours and policies, and engender a spiritual discourse into our humble care and custodianship of natural resources, much as the Kogi have been trying to teach us. My hope is that we do not waste this opportunity and blow the chance to create a revolutionary and emergent dialogue, where all parties can have a say about placing Nature at the core and priority of our forward decision-making processes. Forest bathing is the bridge between these two opposing worlds; it has the ability to bring the magic back into our lives, to unite and inspire.

As practitioners of forest medicine, we have a joyful desire to spread this method of simple reconnection, and my aim is to get every single person on the planet to be out forest bathing – drinking in the *komorebi*,[224] the deep, cool stillness of unfolding being, and sensing that connection between the hoverfly caught momentarily in the shaft of sunlight and the creation of galaxies, right there in that moment of quintessential[225] realisation. I dream of seeing forest bathing as the immediate health intervention for a whole range of issues from insomnia to stress, blood pressure, obesity, and a whole gamut of mental health concerns. Fewer pills, more trees!

Bringing the spiritual and metaphysical into forest bathing is a vital part of our work, without wanting to sound overly proselytising. To make real change in our culture, we need to be brave enough to initiate a new dialogue, a new all-encompassing, interconnected perspective. One where we can entertain some of the ideas from the East – the harmonising principles and some of the Buddhist principles that also see mental processes as being a form of culturally conditioned phenomena.

When we take mindfulness – or my version, mindlessness – into a natural setting, we can begin to appreciate that impermanence is everywhere, and that death, decay, and decomposition are everywhere, and not only part of all natural processes but also mirroring our own inner cycles of growth and decay. Life is transience, and acceptance of this is fundamental. Uncertainty is an aspect of cosmic expression, not achieving a peaceful mind state, but gaining unique insights into the very nature of existence and being, through our ontological enquiries and moments of lucidity.

Meditate on the elements, the seasons, the origin and rebirth of all things, and the gentle observations of the natural world both revealing and reflecting our inner processes, the macro and the micro, and all of life interdependently linked forever both with a start and an end, and without a start or an end, just flowing transforming energy.

My fear is that forest bathing becomes commodified, NVQ-boxed, and relegated to yet another bland, meaningless abstraction, tamed and neutered and absorbed by the milieu of mediocrity and strict compliance, driven by research statistics and outcome measures – blah!

Take to the hills, people, take to the woods, swim in the rivers, challenge the shareholders to be accountable, hold the agencies responsible for our environments and clean water to account, demand quality everywhere, embody wisdom and embrace wilderness in your own lives in a gesture of defiance, and don't forget to notice the beauty all around you, and pass it on to others, to complete strangers.

In that vein, I will end with a wonderfully subversive counterculture poem by environmental activist and poet Wendell Berry.

Manifesto: The Mad Farmer Liberation Front

Love the quick profit, the annual raise,
vacation with pay. Want more
of everything ready-made. Be afraid
to know your neighbors and to die.
And you will have a window in your head.
Not even your future will be a mystery
any more. Your mind will be punched in a card
and shut away in a little drawer.
When they want you to buy something
they will call you. When they want you
to die for profit they will let you know.

So, friends, every day do something
that won't compute. Love the Lord.
Love the world. Work for nothing.
Take all that you have and be poor.
Love someone who does not deserve it.
Denounce the government and embrace
the flag. Hope to live in that free
republic for which it stands.
Give your approval to all you cannot

understand. Praise ignorance, for what man
has not encountered he has not destroyed.

Ask the questions that have no answers.
Invest in the millennium. Plant sequoias.
Say that your main crop is the forest
that you did not plant,
that you will not live to harvest.
Say that the leaves are harvested
when they have rotted into the mold.
Call that profit. Prophesy such returns.

Put your faith in the two inches of humus
that will build under the trees
every thousand years.
Listen to carrion – put your ear
close, and hear the faint chattering
of the songs that are to come.
Expect the end of the world. Laugh.
Laughter is immeasurable. Be joyful
though you have considered all the facts.
So long as women do not go cheap
for power, please women more than men.
Ask yourself: Will this satisfy
a woman satisfied to bear a child?
Will this disturb the sleep
of a woman near to giving birth?

Go with your love to the fields.
Lie down in the shade. Rest your head
in her lap. Swear allegiance
to what is nighest your thoughts.
As soon as the generals and the politicos
can predict the motions of your mind,
lose it. Leave it as a sign
to mark the false trail, the way
you didn't go. Be like the fox
who makes more tracks than necessary,
some in the wrong direction.
Practice resurrection.[226]

References

Introduction: Curlew Dance

1   William James defines 'noetic quality' in this way: 'Although so similar to states of feeling, mystical states seem to those who experience them to be also states of knowledge. They are states of insight into depths of truth unplumbed by the discursive intellect. They are illuminations, revelations, full of significance and importance, all inarticulate though they remain; and as a rule they carry with them a curious sense of authority for after-time.' James, W. (1902) *The Varieties of Religious Experience: A Study in Human Nature*. Longmans, Green & Co.

2   Wareham, T. (2017) *The Green Man of Horam* (self-published); pp. 75–76. Referencing Murray, W. (1946) *Nature's Undiscovered Kingdom*. London: George Allen and Unwin Ltd; p. 46.

3   Wareham, T. (2017) *The Green Man of Horam* (self-published); pp. 75–76. Referencing Murray, W. (1948) *Copsford*; p. 66.

Are We Suffering?

4   Heron, J. (1997) *Helping the Client*. London: SAGE Publications; p. 11.

5   Roszak, T. and Gomes, M.E. (eds) (1995). *Ecopsychology: Restoring the Earth, Healing the Mind*. USA: Counterpoint.

Chapter 1: Aesthetic Ecology

6   Muir, J. (1997) *Nature Writings: The Story of My Boyhood and Youth, My First Summer in the Sierra, the Mountains of California, Stickeen, Selected Essays*. Library of America; p. 814.

7   Hayhow, D.B., Eaton, M.A., Stanbury, A.J., Burns, F., *et al.* (2019) *The State of Nature*. The State of Nature Partnership. Accessed March 2023 at: https://nbn. org.uk/wp-content/uploads/2019/09/State-of-Nature-2019-UK-full-report.pdf.

8   NPK stands for nitrogen, phosphorus, and potassium which are the components of fertiliser.

9   John Muir reminds us that 'God never made an ugly landscape. All that the sun shines on is beautiful, so long as it is wild.' Browning, P. (1988) *John Muir, in His Own Words: A Book of Quotations*. Lafayette: Great West Books.

10 'Ecological writing keeps insisting that we are "embedded" in nature. Nature is a surrounding medium that sustains our being. Due to the properties of the rhetoric that evokes the idea of a surrounding medium, ecological writing can never properly establish that this is nature and thus provide a compelling and consistent

aesthetic basis for the new worldview that is meant to change society. It is a small operation, like tipping over a domino... Putting something called Nature on a pedestal and admiring it from afar does for the environment what patriarchy does for the figure of Woman. It is a paradoxical act of sadistic admiration' Morton, T. (2007) *Ecology without Nature*. Harvard University Press; p. 4–5.

11   The Prince of Wales has now agreed to expand Wistman's Wood following a visit in July 2023.

12   Ulrich, R.S. (1984) View through a window may influence recovery from surgery. *Science* 224, 420–421. https://doi.org/10.1126/science.6143402.

13   Song, C., Ikei, H., and Miyazaki, Y. (2018) Physiological effects of visual stimulation with forest imagery. *Int J Environ Res Public Health* 5, 2, 213. https://doi.org/10.3390/ijerph15020213.

14   Mostajeran, F., Krzikawski, J., Steinicke, F., *et al.* (2021) Effects of exposure to immersive videos and photo slideshows of forest and urban environments. *Sci Rep* 11, 3994. https://doi.org/10.1038/s41598-021-83277-y.

15   Carson, R. (1954) The real world around us. In L. Lear (ed.) (1998) *Lost Woods: The Discovered Writing of Rachel Carson*. Beacon Press.

16   Kazin, A. (ed.) (1979) *The Portable Blake*. London: Penguin Classics.

17   Vazza, F. and Feletti, A. (2017) The Strange Similarity of Neuron and Galaxy Networks. Nautilus Quarterly, July 2017. Accessed July 2023 at https://nautil.us/the-strange-similarity-of-neuron-and-galaxy-networks-236709.

18   Næss, A. (2008) *Ecology of Wisdom*. London: Penguin Random House.

19   Cloos, H. (1953) *Conversation with the Earth*. New York: Knopf.

Consciousness

20   James, W. (1902) *The Varieties of Religious Experience: A Study in Human Nature*. Longmans, Green & Co.

21   The Marginalian (2023). Quoting Challenger, M. (2021) *How to Be Animal: A New History of What it Means to Be Human*. Accessed August 2023 at: www.themarginalian.org/2023/07/10/how-to-be-animal-melanie-challenger.

Chapter 2: The Universe of Nature and the Nature of the Universe

22   Einstein, A. (1936) Extract from a letter to Phyllis Wright.

23   The European Space Agency. Accessed July 2023 at: www.esa.int/Science_Exploration/Space_Science/Planck.

24   Cox, B. and Cohen, A. (2017) *Forces of Nature*. London: William Collins; p.37.

25   Swimme, B. and Berry, T. (1992) *The Universe Story*. New York: HarperCollins; p. 18.

26   Hoyle, F. (1982) The Universe: Past and Present Reflections. *Annual Review of Astronomy and Astrophysics*, 20, 1–36. https://doi.org/10.1146/annurev.aa.20.090182.000245.

27   Ellis, G.F.R. (1993) The Anthropic Principle: Laws and Environments. In: F. Bertola and U.Curi (eds). *The Anthropic Principle*. New York: Cambridge University Press; p. 30.

28   Ward, P. and Brownlee, D.E. (2000) *Rare Earth: Why Complex Life Is Uncommon in the Universe*. New York: Copernicus.

29   Cox, B. and Cohen, A. (2017) *Forces of Nature*. London: William Collins; pp. 97-98.

30   Swimme, B. and Berry, T. (1992) *The Universe Story*. New York: HarperCollins; p. 85.

31   One of Carl Sagan's most famous quotes is: 'The nitrogen in our DNA, the calcium in our teeth, the iron in our blood, the carbon in our apple pies were made in the interiors of collapsing stars. We are made of star stuff.'

32   Cox, B. and Cohen, A. (2017) *Forces of Nature*. London: William Collins; p. 41.

33   The Marginalian. Einstein on Widening Our Circles of Compassion. Accessed July 2023 at: www.themarginalian.org/2016/11/28/einstein-circles-of-compassion.

Beauty and the Bullfinch

34   British Trust for Ornithology (2019). Boom time at Britain's bird feeders. www.bto.org/press-releases/boom-time-britains-bird-feeders.

Chapter 3: Nature, Philosophy, and Disconnection

35   Aristotle. *Metaphysics*. 983: b6; 8–11.

36   Aristotle. *De Anima*. 411: a7–8.

37   Another Greek word originating from this time is *physis* which means 'nature' or 'essence', and translates into Latin as *natura*. *Physis* is the origin of the science of physics, which means 'to be born' or 'to emerge into being'.

38   The Japanese call this *ikigai*, meaning 'reason for being', 'life purpose', or 'bliss': it's about the passion for being alive, in full possession of one's life joy and expression.

39   In Ancient Greek cosmogony it was believed that the Universe was born from *Chaos*, a mythological void, or primordial state that preceded the creation of the Universe and the first gods. Chaos may refer to a limitless space and formless matter stretching to infinity.

40   King James Bible. Genesis, 1:2.

41   MacDonell, A.A. (2006) *Hymns from the Rigveda*. Read Books. 10; 129:6.

42   The term 'quantum mechanics' was first coined in the early 1920s by a group of physicists including Max Born based at Göttingen University, Germany. Among those scientists working on quantum theory were Werner Heisenberg, Erwin Schrödinger, and Neils Bohr. These three had a deep interest in Eastern philosophy and the *Upanishads*, the Vedanta or last of the Vedic texts that form the basis of Hindu philosophy.

43   Capra, F. (1988) *Uncommon Wisdom*. Shambhala; p. 43.

44   Capra, F. (2010) *The Tao of Physics*. Shambhala.

45   Schrödinger, E. (1974) *What Is Life?* Cambridge University Press; Epilogue.

46   Schrödinger, E. (1974) *What Is Life?* Cambridge University Press; Epilogue.

47   Schrödinger, E. (1951) *My View of the World*. Cambridge University Press.

48   Park, D. (2005) *The Grand Contraption*. Princeton University Press.

49   Lao Tzu (1972) *Tao Te Ching*. Trans. Ch'u Ta-kao. Allen & Unwin. Ch II; p. 13.

50   Lao Tzu (1972) *Tao Te Ching*. Trans. Ch'u Ta-kao. Allen & Unwin. Ch LI; p. 66.

51   King James Bible. Genesis, 2:7.

52   'And it seems to me that that which possessed thought is what people call air, and that by this everyone both is governed and has power over everything. For it is this which seems to me to be god and to have reached everything and to arrange everything and to be in everything. And there is not a single thing which does not share in it.' (Burnet. J. (1930) *Simplicius On Aristotle*, Physics p. 151, 24. London: A&C Black; p. 353)

53 Capra, F. and Luisi P.L. (2014) *The Systems View of Life*. Cambridge University Press; p. 5.

54 Plato. *Timaeus*. Trans. W.R.M. Lamb (1925).

55 Lovelock, J.E. and Margulis, L. (1974). Atmospheric homeostasis by and for the biosphere: the gaia hypothesis. *Tellus*, 26: 1-2, 2–10. doi: 10.3402/tellusa.v26i1-2.9731.

56 Oxford Online Dictionary. Inspire. Accessed July 2023 at: www.oxfordlearners-dictionaries.com/definition/english/inspire?q=inspire.

57 Abram, D. (1996) *The Spell of the Sensuous*. New York: Vintage Books; p. 117.

58 Plato. *Phaedrus Dialogues*. 230d.

59 Capra F. (2010) *The Tao of Physics*. Shambhala; p. 257.

Poetry

60 Santayana, G. (1990) The elements and function of poetry. In: *Interpretations of Poetry and Religion*. MIT Press; p. 278.

Chapter 4: *Phantasiai*: Philosophy, Mysticism, and Reconnection

61 For more detail on this topic, I direct the reader towards David Abram's excellent book *The Spell of the Sensuous*.

62 As quoted in Lachapelle, D. (1992) *Sacred Land, Sacred Sex – The Rapture of the Deep*. Durango, CO: Kivaki Press; p. 23.

63 Plato. *Timaeus*. (90a-b)

64 Lawrence, D.H. (1930) *A Propos for Lady Chatterley's Lover*. London: Mandrake Press.

65 Schopenhauer, A. (1819) *The World as Will and Idea*. Vol. II, Ch. XLVIII. www.gutenberg.org/ebooks/38427.

66 Robbins, B.D. (2006) The delicate empiricism of Goethe: Phenomenology as a rigorous science of nature. *Indo-Pacific Journal of Phenomenology 6*, suppl 1, 1–13. https://doi.org/10.1080/20797222.2006.11433928.

67 As quoted in Wood, J. (1893) *Dictionary of Quotations from Ancient and Modern, English and Foreign Sources*. 183: 24.

68 Barrows, A. and Macey, J. (1996) *Rilke's Book of Hours: Love Poems to God*. New York: Riverhead Books; pp. 1, 45.

69 The economy of Rilke's writing reminds me of the American Zen Buddhist poet Gary Snyder. Snyder has had a massive impact on my life and how I made sense of some of my Nature experiences. Snyder's style, shorn of extraneous words, sparse and pure like haiku, was often the tonic I needed in my search for meaning. His slightly irreverent poetry won't be to everyone's taste, but his observations of life are so powerful.

70 Wordsworth, W. (1798) 'Lines Composed a Few Miles above Tintern Abbey, On Revisiting the Banks of the Wye during a Tour, July 13, 1798.'

71 Marcus Aurelius. *Meditations*, iv. 40.

72 Rather than trying to re-invent the wheel, I refer you to the excellent book by Tom Wareham called *The Green Man of Horam* (2017) about the life and writings of Walter Murray. It is the perfect appraisal of this process of revelation, realisation and wonderment towards Nature.

73 Jefferies, R. (1909) The Pageant of Summer. In: Thomas, E. (ed). *The Life of the Fields*. London: Duckworth; pp. 270–279.

74 James, W. (1902) *The Varieties of Religious Experience: A Study in Human Nature*. Longmans, Green & Co.

75 Wareham, T. (2017) *The Green Man of Horam* (self-published); p. 106. Referencing Murray, W. (1950) 'Nature Notes April 1950'.

76 Oliver, M. (1986) 'Wild Geese'. In: *Dream Work*. New York: Grove Atlantic.

77 A reference to one of Walter Murray's best books, *Nature's Undiscovered Kingdom* (1947). London: George Allen & Unwin.

78 Wareham, T. (2017) *The Green Man of Horam* (self-published); p. 80. Referencing Murray, W. (1950) *Nature's Undiscovered Kingdom*.

79 Wareham, T. (2017) *The Green Man of Horam* (self-published); p. 103. Referencing Murray, W. (1950) *Nature's Undiscovered Kingdom*.

80 James, W. (1902) *The Varieties of Religious Experience: A Study in Human Nature*. James identified four main characteristics of a mystical experience: Ineffability, a Noetic quality, Transience, and Passivity.

81 Wareham, T. (2017) *The Green Man of Horam* (self-published); p. 95. Referencing Mercer, J.E. (1912) *Nature Mysticism*; p. 169.

Thuggery

82 World Economic Forum (2019). 'Our house is on fire.' 16 year-old Greta Thunberg wants action. Accessed August 2023 at: www.weforum.org/agenda/2019/01/our-house-is-on-fire-16-year-old-greta-thunberg-speaks-truth-to-power.

83 On a positive note, Harvard experimental psychologist Steven Pinker argues that despite our instinctive pessimism, we are, according to data, becoming less violent as a species in his book *The Better Angels of Our Nature* (2011).

84 Lanier, J. (2011) *You Are Not a Gadget*. London: Penguin Books; p. 75.

85 For those who would like to read more on this topic, I highly recommend Jeremy Lent's excellent book *The Patterning Instinct: A Cultural History of Humanity's Search for Meaning* (2017), New York: Prometheus.

86 'All streams flow to the sea because it is lower than they are. Humility gives it its power. If you want to govern the people, you must place yourself below them. If you want to lead the people, you must learn how to follow them.' Lao Tzu, *Tao Te Ching*.

87 Anderson, R. (2021) *The Divine Feminine Tao Te Ching*. Vermont: Inner Traditions.

88 9th Debate. Sanders Theatre, Harvard Museum of Natural History. September 2009.

89 Lent, J. (2017) *The Patterning Instinct: A Cultural History of Humanity's Search for Meaning*. New York: Prometheus; p. 141.

90 Capra, F. (2010) *The Tao of Physics*. Boulder, CO: Shambhala.

Chapter 5: Oriental Philosophy

91 Neither are technically religions in the sense that there is no single diety or dogmas.

92 Scroope, C. (2021) Japanese Culture. Religion. Accessed July 2023 at: https://culturalatlas.sbs.com.au/japanese-culture/japanese-culture-religion.

93 Manabu, T. (2017) Nature Worship in Old Shintō. Accessed July 2023 at: www.nippon.com/en/views/b05213/.

94 Rots, A.P. (2017) *Shinto, Nature and Ideology in Contemporary Japan*. London and New York: Bloomsbury Academic.

95 Rots, A.P. (2017) *Shinto, Nature and Ideology in Contemporary Japan*. London and New York: Bloomsbury Academic; p. 94.

96 Rots, A.P. (2017) *Shinto, Nature and Ideology in Contemporary Japan*. London and New York: Bloomsbury Academic; p. 95.

97 Wong, E. (2011) *Taoism: An Essential Guide*. Boston: Shambhala; p. 22.

98 Zhang, J. (2001) 'A Declaration of the Chinese Daoist Association on Global Ecology'. In Girardot, N.J., Miller, J. and Xiaogan, L. (eds.). *Daoism and Ecology: Ways Within a Cosmic Landscape*. Cambridge, MA: Center for the Study of World Religions.

99 Terry and Larry are the authors of this piece. Terrie and Larry live half the year in Portal, Arizona, where they have had twelve species of hummingbird at their feeders. The rest of the year they are in Pawleys Island, SC, where they enjoy Ruby-throated Hummingbirds and once had a Rufous Hummingbird.

100 Lao Tzu (1972) *Tao Te Ching*. Trans. Ch'u Ta-kao. Allen & Unwin; Chapter 10.

101 Please see also the following two excellent books: *Tao: The Watercourse Way* by Alan Watts (2019, Souvenir Press) which is full of interesting insights alongside beautiful calligraphy representing the flow of water; and *The Tao of Leadership* by John Heider (2015, Green Dragon Books), which updates Lao Tzu's original advice for modern leaders.

Why?

102 Thoreau, H.D. (1854) *Walden; or, Life in the Woods.*

103 Snyder, G. (2013) 'Remaining Unprepared'. The Hopwood lecture at The University of Michigan, April 24 2013.

104 Feynman, R. P. (2008). *Perfectly Reasonable Deviations from the Beaten Track: The Letters of Richard P. Feynman*. Hachette UK; p. 256.

Chapter 6: Fundamentals of *Shinrin-Yoku*

105 https://natureandtherapy.co.uk.

106 Miyazaki, Y. (2007) *Science of Natural Therapy*. Chiba: Chiba University. https://smartcdn.gprod.postmedia.digital/vancouversun/wp-content/uploads/2010/08/naturaltherapy.pdf.

107 The World Bank. Forest Area (% of Land Area) – Japan. Accessed July 2023 at: https://data.worldbank.org/indicator/AG.LND.FRST.ZS?locations=JP.

108 Hemery, G. European Countries and Their Forest Cover. Accessed July 2023 at: https://gabrielhemery.com/european-countries-and-their-forest-cover/.

109 World Health Organization. (2022) Ambient (Outdoor) Air Pollution. Accessed July 2023 at: www.who.int/news-room/fact-sheets/detail/ambient-(outdoor)-air-quality-and-health.

110 World Economic Forum. (2022) This Chart Shows the Impact Rising Urbanization Will Have on the World. Accessed July 2023 at: www.weforum.org/agenda/2022/04/global-urbanization-material-consumption/.

111 Miyazaki, Y., Ikei, H., and Song, C. (2014) [Forest medicine research in Japan]. *Nihon Eiseigaku Zasshi, 69*, 2, 122–135. doi: 10.1265/jjh.69.122.

112 Miyazaki, Y., Ikei, H., and Song, C. (2014) [Forest medicine research in Japan]. *Nihon Eiseigaku Zasshi 69*, 2, 122–135. https://doi.org/10.1265/jjh.69.122.

113 Kaplan, R. and Kaplan, S. (1989) *The Experience of Nature: A Psychological Perspective*. Cambridge University Press.

114 Kabat-Zinn, J. (2010) *Coming to Our Senses*. London: Piatkus; p. 108.

115 Capra, F. and Luisi, P.L. (2014) *The Systems View of Life*. Cambridge: Cambridge University Press; pp. 64–68. For further detail on this fascinating topic, I refer the reader to this excellent and complex work by Fritjof Capra and Pier Luigi Luisi.

Relationship, Reciprocity, The Dance

116 Oliver, M. (1990) 'Summer day'. In: *House of Light*. Beacon Press

117 Eliot, T.S. (1935) 'Burnt Norton'. *Collected Poems 1909–1962*. New York: Harcourt, Brace & World.

Chapter 7: Health

118 The word mother originates from the Sanskrit *Mātr* which means 'one who gave birth' and also derives from a root word meaning 'that which is respected' (the word matrix also comes from the same Sanskrit root and means 'uterus or womb'). The term Earth-Mother has been in common use since at least the 1580s.

119 Wizards are 'wise-ards'. The word witch has long been associated with negative connotations but derives from Old English and Anglo-Saxon words *Wicca* and *Wicce* which variously translate as 'divinatory', 'sorceress', and also in an early translation of the Bible as 'midwife'.

120 I particularly dislike the three words in bold. 'Sustainability' indicates that we can carry on as before by adjusting a few things, e.g., get an electric SUV, and similarly 'resilience' suggests that if we incorporate some self-care practices into our lives, we can carry on stronger. We should not be strong! We should be very sensitive and easily hurt by the damage that things are doing to us. Finally, 'sit-spot' feels like a derogatory casual term for a beautiful activity borrowed from First Nations culture. Please find a new term for this sacred activity!

121 Evans, K. (2020) The New Zealand river that became a legal person. Accessed February 2023 at: www.bbc.com/travel/article/20200319-the-new-zealand-river-that-became-a-legal-person.

122 Whitburn, J., Linklater, W., and Abrahamse, W. (2020) Meta-analysis of human connection to nature and proenvironmental behavior. *Conservation Biology* 34, 1, 180–193.

123 Deci, E.L. and Ryan, R.M. (2012) Self-determination theory. In: Van Lange, P.A.M., Kruglanski, A.W., and Higgins E.T. (eds) *Handbook of Theories of Social Psychology*. Sage Publications Ltd; pp. 416–436. https://doi.org/10.4135/9781446249215.n21.

124 Abraham Maslow's hierarchy of needs (1943) is a motivational theory in psychology presuming a universal set of survival motives. These are represented as a five-tier model of human needs, often depicted as hierarchical levels within a pyramid diagram. The needs lower down in the hierarchy must be satisfied before individuals can attend to needs higher up. From the bottom of the hierarchy upwards, they are: physiological, safety, love and belonging, esteem, and self-actualisation at the top of the pyramid.

125 Griffin, J. and Tyrrell, I. (1998) The 'human givens'. *The Therapist*, 5, 1, 24–29. See also: www.hgi.org.uk.

Chapter 9: Thresholds

126 O'Donohue, J. (2008) *To Bless the Space Between Us*. Boulder, CO: Convergent Books.

127 Cousin, G. (2006) An introduction to threshold concepts. *Planet 17*, December 2006, 4–5.

128 Oxford English Dictionary. Liminality. Accessed August 2023 at: www.oed.com/search/advanced/Entries?q=liminality&sortOption=Frequency.

129 van Gennep, A. (1977). *The Rites of Passage*. Routledge & Kegan Paul; p. 21.

130 Meyer, J.H.F., Land R., and Baillie, C. (eds) (2010) *Threshold Concepts and Transformational Learning*. Rotterdam: Sense Publishers; pp. ix–xiii.

131 Szakolczai, A. (2009) Liminality and experience: structuring transitory situations and transformative events. *International Political Anthropology 2* , 1, 141–172.

132 Turner, V. (1967) *The Forest of Symbols*. Ithaca, NY: Cornell University Press.

133 Thomassen, B. (2009) The uses and meanings of liminality. *International Political Anthropology 2*, 1, 5–27.

134 This term has come to be applied recently in connection with the surge in psychedelic medicine events which may also integrate the three-stage liminality process.

135 O'Donohue, J. (2008) *To Bless the Space Between Us*. Boulder, CO: Convergent Books.

Nature as Lover, Paramour

136 Shepherd, N. (2008) *The Living Mountain*. Edinburgh: Canongate.

Chapter 10: A Polyphony of The Senses

137 Shepherd, N. (2008) *The Living Mountain*. Edinburgh: Canongate; p. 104.

138 Wedekind, C., Seebeck, T., Bettens, F., and Paepke, A.J. (1995) MHC-dependent mate preferences in humans. *Proceedings of the Royal Society of London 260*, 1359, 245–249. https://doi.org/10.1098/rspb.1995.0087.

139 Chodorow, J. (2014) The History and Multi-Sensory Nature of Active Imagination. Accessed August 2023 at: https://ipacamp.org.br/the-history-and-multi-sensory-nature-of-active-imagination.

140 Young, J.Z. (1968) Influence of the mouth on the evolution of the brain. In: Person, P. (ed.) *Biology of the Mouth*. Washington, DC: American Association for the Advancement of Science; pp. 21–35.

141 Bucci, R. (2019) Sometimes when we touch. Accessed December 2023 at: https://brainworldmagazine.com/sometimes-when-we-touch/.

142 Pallasmaa, J. (2005) *The Eyes of the Skin*, 2nd edition. New Jersey: John Wiley and Sons.

143 Jung, C.G., as quoted in Sabini, M. (ed.) (2008) *The Earth Has a Soul*. Berkeley, CA: North Atlantic Books.

144 Shepherd, N. (2008) *The Living Mountain*. Edinburgh: Canongate.

145 Jung, C.J. (1976) *Visions. Seminars Vol. 2*. New York: Spring Publications; p. 473.

146 Pallasmaa, J. (2005) *The Eyes of the Skin*, 2nd edition. New Jersey: John Wiley and Sons.

147 Pallasmaa, J. (2005) *The Eyes of the Skin*, 2nd edition. New Jersey: John Wiley and Sons; p. 58.

148 'The importance of touch can't be understated,' says Dr Matt Hertenstein, an experimental psychologist at Indiana's DePauw University. 'We see touch develop as one of the first modalities when the baby is in the mother's womb. It is our very first connection to the world,' says Hertenstein. 'It takes precedence early and never leaves us.' When we are touched, or when we touch something or someone, pressure receptors under the skin send signals to the brain, which responds by undergoing a series of physiological reactions. (Bucci, R. (2019) Sometimes when we touch. Accessed December 2023 at: https://brainworldmagazine.com/sometimes-when-we-touch/.)

149 Marais, A., Adams, B., Ringsmuth, A.K., Ferretti, M., *et al.* (2018) The future of quantum biology. *Journal of the Royal Society Interface, 15*, 20180640. http://doi.org/10.1098/rsif.2018.0640.

150 Torgan. C. (2014) Humans can identity more than 1 trillion smells. Accessed December 2023 at: www.nih.gov/news-events/nih-research-matters/humans-can-identify-more-1-trillion-smells.

151 Powell, M. (n.d.) Is cleaner air killing the Scouse accent? Accessed December 2023 at: www.dailymail.co.uk/health/article-25752/Is-cleaner-air-killing-Scouse-accent.html.

152 Krusemark, E.A., Novak, L.R., Gitelman, D.R., and Li, W. (2013) When the sense of smell meets emotion: anxiety-state-dependent olfactory processing and neural circuitry adaptation. *Journal of Neuroscience 33*, 39, 15324–15332. https://doi.org/10.1523/JNEUROSCI.1835-13.2013.

153 Sheldrake, M. (2020) *Entangled Life*. The Bodley Head; pp. 232–233.

154 National Institutes of Health (2016) How does our sense of taste work? Accessed December 2023 at: www.ncbi.nlm.nih.gov/books/NBK279408/.

155 People used to believe that all music came from birds, that they somehow gave birth to musical sounds or notes, which I really like, especially as a small flock of great tits are all calling each other in the hedge outside my window.

156 Berendt, J.E. (1991) *The World is Sound*. Rochester, VT: Nada Brahma Destiny Books; p. 135.

157 National Institutes of Health (2015) How do we hear? Accessed August 2023 at: www.nidcd.nih.gov/health/how-do-we-hear.

158 'A starting point for me was my interest in hearing, my experience that modern human beings have lost themselves in such a hypertrophy of the visual that they no longer are able to listen adequately. I had wanted to write a book about listening, but – to my initial surprise – it turned out to be a spiritual book. The deterioration of our sense of hearing has run remarkably parallel with the process of secularisation...modern human beings no longer listen.' (Berendt, J.E. (1991) *The World is Sound*. Rochester, VT: Nada Brahma Destiny Books; p. 6.)

159 Merleau-Ponty, M. (2002) *The Phenomenology of Perception*. Abingdon: Routledge Classics; p. 142.

160 Pallasmaa, J. (2005) *The Eyes of the Skin*, 2nd edition. New Jersey: John Wiley and Sons; p. 22.

161 de Certeau, M. (2011) *The Practice of Everyday Life*. University of California Press Books.

162 Bernays, E. (1928) *Propaganda*. New York: Horace Liveright.

163 Pallasmaa, J. (2005) *The Eyes of the Skin*, 2nd edition. New Jersey: John Wiley and Sons.

164 Kaplan, S. (1995) The restorative benefits of nature: Toward an integrative framework. *Journal of Environmental Psychology, 15*, 169–182.

165 Huxley, A. (1943) *The Art of Seeing*. London: Chatto and Windus; p.16.

166 Blake, W. (1790) *The Marriage of Heaven and Hell*. Plate 14.

167 Huxley, A. (1955) Letter to Dr. H. Osmond. In: *Moksha* (1983) Penguin Books; p. 109.

168 Pallasmaa, J. (2005) *The Eyes of the Skin*, 2nd edition. New Jersey: John Wiley and Sons.

169 Zahn, J. (1687) System der visuellen Wahrnehmung beim Menschen. Illustration depicting Emission theory. Accessed August 2023 at: https://commons.wikimedia.org/wiki/File:Fotothek_df_tg_0001920_Optik_%5E_Anatomie_%5E_Mensch_%5E_Auge.jpg.

170 Descartes; Diagram of ocular refraction. Accessed December 2023 at: https://commons.wikimedia.org/wiki/File:Descartes;_Diagram_of_ocular_refraction._Wellcome_L0012003.jpg.

171 Merleau-Ponty, M. (2002) *Phenomenology of Perception*. London: Psychology Press; p. 12.

172 Jung, C. The Psychology of Transference. In: *Collected Works* 16, par. 492.

Simulacra

173 Kellner, D. (1987) Baudrillard, semiurgy and death. *Theory, Culture & Society*, 4, 1, 125–146. https://doi.org/10.1177/026327687004001007.

Chapter 11: Phytoncides and Trees

174 'The Blue Mountains are densely populated by oil bearing Eucalyptus trees. The atmosphere is filled with finely dispersed droplets of oil, which, in combination with dust particles and water vapour, scatter short-wave length rays of light which are predominantly blue in colour.' Accessed August 2023 at: www.bluemts.com.au/info/about/history/history-detail.

175 Went, F. (1960) Blue hazes in the atmosphere. *Nature 187*, 641–643. https://doi.org/10.1038/187641a0.

176 Gordon, H. and Scott, C. (2016) Trees are much better at creating clouds and cooling the climate than we thought. Accessed August 2023 at: https://theconversation.com/trees-are-much-better-at-creating-clouds-and-cooling-the-climate-than-we-thought-66713.

177 Both have written books on *shinrin-yoku* and have contributed to over a hundred research papers which are available online.

178 McKay, J. (dir.) (2016) *Call of the Forest: The Forgotten Wisdom of Trees*. Merit Motion Pictures and Edgeland Films.

179 Salehi, B., Upadhyay, S., Erdogan Orhan, I., Kumar Jugran, A., *et al.* (2019) Therapeutic potential of α- and β-pinene: a miracle gift of nature. *Biomolecules 14*, 9(11), 738. https://doi.org/10.3390/biom9110738.

180 Guenther, A.B., Jiang, X., Heald, C.L., Sakulyanontvittaya, T., *et al.* (2012) The Model of Emissions of Gases and Aerosols from Nature version 2.1 (MEGAN2.1): an extended and updated framework for modeling biogenic emissions. *Geoscientific Model Development 5*, 1471–1492. https://doi.org/10.5194/gmd-5-1471-2012.

181 'The quirks of quantum physics are something you might expect to find under exotic conditions in a laboratory, but not in a meadow. Yet in recent years, a

blossoming idea called quantum biology proposes that life's molecular mechanisms deploy some of those notoriously counterintuitive behaviours. Ten years ago, researchers reported evidence that photosynthesis – the process by which green plants and some bacteria turn sunlight into chemical energy – gains light-harvesting efficiency by exploiting the phenomenon of "quantum coherence". This involves the superpositions of electronic quantum states, which seem able to explore many energy-transmitting pathways at once. If so, quantum mechanics is assisting the fundamental energetic process that drives all life on the surface of the Earth.' (Ball, P. (2018) Is photosynthesis quantum-ish? https://physicsworld.com/a/is-photosynthesis-quantum-ish.)

182 Roviello, V. and Roviello, G.N. (2020) Lower COVID-19 mortality in Italian forested areas suggests immunoprotection by Mediterranean plants. *Environmental Chemistry Letters* 19, 699–710. https://doi.org/10.1007/s10311-020-01063-0.

Chapter 12: Risk

183 Keller, H. (1946) *Let Us Have Faith*. Garden City, NY: Doubleday & Company; pp. 50–51.

184 Bargh, J. (1994) *The Preconscious in Social Interactions*. Washington: American Psychological Society, as quoted in Goleman, D. (1996) *Emotional Intelligence*. London: Bloomsbury Publishing; p. 20.

185 Cairns, W. (2008) *How to Live Dangerously: Why We Should All Stop Worrying, and Start Living*. London: Macmillan; p. x.

186 Watt, J. and Ball, D.J. (2009) Trees and the risk of harm. Accessed August 2023 at: https://ntsgroup.org.uk/wp-content/uploads/2016/06/NTSG-Report-1_Trees-and-the-Risk-of-Harm.pdf.

187 Mortlock, C. (1998) *The Adventure Alternative*. Cumbria, UK: Cicerone Press.

188 Macfarlane, R. (2009) *Mountains of the Mind*. London: Granta Books.

189 Hoff, B. (1983) *The Tao of Pooh*. London: Penguin Books.

Chapter 13: The Savage Self

190 Midgeley, M. (2002) *Beast and Man*. Oxford: Routledge; p. xxxiii.

191 Kellert, S.R. and Wilson, E.O. (1993) *The Biophilia Hypothesis*. Washington, DC: Island Press.

192 Selhuba E. and Logan, A. (2014) *Your Brain on Nature*. Toronto, ON: Harper Collins.

193 Ulrich, R.S. (1984) View through a window may influence recovery from surgery. Accessed December 2023 at: https://lebonheurestdanslejardin.files.wordpress.com/2019/06/ulrich-1984.pdf.

194 Cregan-Reid, V. (2018) *Primate Change*. London: Octopus; pp. 16–17.

195 Kellert, S.R. and Wilson, E.O. (1993) *The Biophilia Hypothesis*. Washington, DC: Island Press; p. 32.

196 Deleuze, G. and Guattari, F. (1983) *Anti-Oedipus: Capitalism and Schizophrenia*. Minneapolis, MN: University of Minnesota Press.

197 Huxley, A. (1954) *The Doors of Perception*. London: Chatto and Windus.

198 Mayer, E.A. (2011) Gut feelings: the emerging biology of gut-brain communication. *Nature Reviews Neuroscience* 12, 8, 453–466. https://doi.org/10.1038/nrn3071.

199 Liu, L., Huh, J.R., and Shah, K. (2022) Microbiota and the gut-brain-axis: Implications for new therapeutic design in the CNS. *EBioMedicine, 77*, 103908. https://doi.

org/10.1016/j.ebiom.2022.103908. (See also the NIH Human Microbiome Project at: https://hmpdacc.org.)

200 Kelly, J.R., Kennedy, P.J., Cryan, J.F., Dinan, T.G., Clarke, G., and Hyland, N.P. (2015) Breaking down the barriers: the gut microbiome, intestinal permeability and stress-related psychiatric disorders. *Frontiers in Cell Neuroscience 9*, 392. https://doi.org/10.3389/fncel.2015.00392.

201 Rogers, G., Keating, D., Young, R. *et al.* (2016) From gut dysbiosis to altered brain function and mental illness: mechanisms and pathways. *Molecular Psychiatry 21*, 738–748. https://doi.org/10.1038/mp.2016.50.

202 'Descartes' dualism also forms the basis for the modern view of our relationship with the natural world... With this step, Descartes completed the process, begun by monotheism, that eliminated any intrinsic value from the natural world. With nothing sacred about nature, it became available for the human intellect to use remorselessly for its own purposes.' (Lent, J. (2017) *The Patterning Instinct*. New York: Prometheus Books; p. 237.)

203 Midgley, M. (2002) *Beast and Man*. London: Routledge; p. 39.

204 Sokolowski, K. and Corbin, J.G. (2012) Wired for behaviors: from development to function of innate limbic system circuitry. *Frontiers in Molecular Neuroscience 5*, 55. https://doi.org/10.3389/fnmol.2012.00055.

205 Diogo, R., Siomava, N., and Gitton, Y. (2019) Development of human limb muscles based on whole-mount immunostaining and the links between ontogeny and evolution. *Development 146*, 20: dev180349.

206 Deleuze, G. (1991) *Bergsonism*. New York: Zone Books; p. 13.

207 Wikipedia. Intuition. Accessed August 2023 at: https://en.wikipedia.org/wiki/Intuition.

208 Jung, C. (1970) *Man and His Symbols*. New York: Dell Publishing; p. 49.

209 Maritain, J. (1953) *Creative Intuition in Art and Poetry*. Bollingen Foundation.

210 Jung, C.G., as quoted in Sabini, M. (ed.) (2008) *The Earth Has a Soul*. Berkeley, CA: North Atlantic Books; p. 19.

211 Jung, C.G. (1940) Modern Psychology. Lecture at ETH Zurich Dec. 20th 1940. In: *Alchemy*. Bollingen Princeton University Press; Lecture VII, p. 67.

212 Jung, C.J. (1977) *Interviews and Encounters*. McGuire, W. and Hull, R.F.C. (eds). Princeton University Press; p.57.

213 Jung, C.G., as quoted in Sabini, M. (ed.) (2008) *The Earth Has a Soul*. Berkeley, CA: North Atlantic Books; p. 16.

214 Bleakley, A. (1988) *Fruits of the Moon Tree*. Bath: Gateway Books.

215 Jung, C.G., as quoted in Sabini, M. (ed.) (2008) *The Earth Has a Soul*. Berkeley, CA: North Atlantic Books.

216 Monbiot, G. (2013) *Feral*. London: Penguin Books; p. 34.

217 Bleakley, A. (1988) *Fruits of the Moon Tree*. Bath: Gateway Books; p. 155.

218 Carson, R. (1954) *Exceeding Beauty of the Earth*. Talk given to women journalists, Columbus, Ohio US, 21 April 1954.

Chapter 14: Lost

219 Murat Ildan, M. (2021) *Aforizmalar* [Aphorisms]. Istanbul: Siyah Beyaz Publishing House. https://muratildanquotations.wordpress.com.

220 Muir, J. As quoted in Palmer, A.W. (1911) *The Mountain Trail and Its Message*. Boston: Pilgrim Press.

221 Wagoner, D. (1966) *Staying Alive*. Indianapolis University Press.

222 Wagoner, D. (1972) 'Lost'. In: *Riverbed*. Indiana University Press.

Chapter 15: Conclusions

223 For more detail on this, please read the excellent *The Heart of the World* (1990) by Alan Ereira.
224 See section on *komorebi* in Chapter 1, Aesthetic Ecology.
225 Quintessence = fifth element of life.
226 Berry, W. (2018) *The Peace of Wild Things*. London: Penguin Random House.

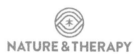

NATURE & THERAPY

The International Forest Therapy Diploma is a 3-stage accredited qualification in *shinrin-yoku* (forest bathing). The course is run from Devon and other venues throughout the year. See website for details www.natureandtherapy.co.uk